Caring in Crisis

An Oral History of Critical Care Nursing

Jacqueline Zalumas

University of Pennsylvania Press

Philadelphia

dlc

Permission is acknowledged to reprint materials from published sources:

"Nick: A Case Study," from Dolores M. Garlo, "Critical Care Nurses: A Case for Legal Recognition of the Growing Responsibilities and Accountability in the Nursing Profession," *Journal of Contemporary Law* 11(1) (1984): 239–285. Copyright © 1984 by the *Journal of Contemporary Law*. Reprinted by permission of the author and the *Journal of Contemporary Law*, University of Utah College of Law.

Table 1, "Domains of Nursing Practice and Identified Competencies," from P. Benner, *From Novice to Expert: Excellence and Power in Clinical Nursing Practice* (Menlo Park, CA: Addison-Wesley, 1984). Copyright © 1984 by Addison-Wesley Publishing Company. Used by permission of the author and Addison-Wesley Publishing Company.

Library of Congress Cataloging-in-Publication Data

Zalumas, Jacqueline.
   Caring in crisis : an oral history of critical care nursing / Jacqueline Zalumas.
      p.   cm. — (University of Pennsylvania Press studies in health, illness, and caregiving)
   Includes bibliographical references and index.
   ISBN 0-8122-3255-0 (cloth). — ISBN 0-8122-1510-9 (pbk.)
   1. Intensive care nursing — United States — History. 2. Oral history. 3. Nurses — United States — Interviews. I. Title. II. Series: Studies in health, illness, and caregiving.
   [DNLM: 1. History of Nursing — United States. 2. Critical Care — history — United States. WY 11 AA1 Z2c 1994]
RT120.I5Z35   1994
610.73'61 — dc20
DNLM/DLC
for Library of Congress   94-22352
                                                                                       CIP

Caring in Crisis

University of Pennsylvania Press
STUDIES IN HEALTH, ILLNESS, AND CAREGIVING
Joan E. Lynaugh, General Editor

A list of the books
in the series appears at the
back of this volume

*This book is dedicated to
critical care nurses and their patients.*

This is their story.

I have tried to identify this thing that everybody who is a nurse does, and how the service you give to our society could be phrased. It seems to me that you protect all those who are or who could be in danger from illness, from strain, from shock, from fatigue, from sorrow, from grief; that every spot in this society where there are those who are in danger and who need continuous concern, this is the place where you might function.

Margaret Mead, 1956

Contents

Acknowledgments

This book began with my gradual realization of the invisibility of nurses and nursing practice in the history of health care. The absence of the richness of the experience of nurses with patients in histories is similar to the anonymity of women in written histories. This idea matured into a focused study of the development of critical care nursing. An endeavor that grows as this one did, using oral history methods, is not accomplished alone. Many individuals very generously and graciously contributed to the dissertation research at Emory University that was the foundation of this book. The late Fred R. Crawford, Professor of Sociology, was the first to share with me his vision of the significance of the voices of ordinary people in extraordinary circumstances in revealing the human spirit. The late Jack S. Boozer, Charles Howard Candler Professor of Religion, Emeritus, and David R. Blumenthal, Professor of Religion, both nurtured that interest and encouraged the development of critical thinking essential to the accomplishment of scholarly research. Solomon Sutker, Adjunct Professor of Sociology, supported me through this effort with his friendship, his caring, and his scholarly criticism. The advice of Allen Tullos, Associate Professor, American Studies, Institute of Liberal Arts, to "let the interviews tell the story" was the guiding force behind the interpretation and writing. LaRetta Garland, Professor of Nursing, Emeritus, and Elizabeth Stevenson, Charles Howard Candler Professor of American Studies, Emeritus, gave generously of their time and skills, both during the original research and through later revisions.

Oral history requires technical expertise and resources. I have been blessed with both. Steve Ellwood and Corky Gallo, Media Department, Nell Hodgson Woodruff School of Nursing, Emory University, offered valuable technical support in planning and executing the interviews. Their advice on audiotape software, instrumentation, and variables affecting sound quality greatly enhanced the quality of the taped interviews with critical care nurses. Marilyn Eckstine showed both her friendship to me and her expertise in administration through her efforts in obtaining skilled assistance for transcribing the twenty-five interviews.

Joan Lynaugh, Ph.D., FAAN, Professor, School of Nursing, and Director, Center for the Study of the History of Nursing, University of Pennsylvania, believed in the possibility that these stories of critical care nurses would be told. She provided encouragement, professional guidance, and spirited advice in the writing. I thank her.

Diligent editing, encouragement, and critiques were provided by many friends and professional colleagues. I thank Rose Cannon, MN, RN; Sylvia Fields, RN, Ed.D.; Lisbet Makonnen, RN; John Merriman, MA; Helen O'Shea, RN, Ph.D.; Solomon Sutker, Ph.D.; and Virginia Zalumas. Many others have shown, generosity and caring support in so many specific ways. I especially thank LuRae Ahrendt, RN; Rick Bass, RN; Donna Boles, RN; Wanda Cooper, RN, MN; Maggie Gilead, RN, Ph.D.; Michelle Gray, RN, MN; Barbara Harris, RN, MN; Megan Hawkins, RN; Jo Ann Hollingsworth, RN, MN; Linda Levinson RN; Richard Levinson, Ph.D.; Lynn McIntyre; Jean Ortiz Pruitt, RN, MN; Linda Roberts, DSN, RN; Cama Sell, RN; Carol Simon, RN, Pharm.D. (Simon and Macintosh); Cara Thornly; Angie Whitlow; and Gigi Whitlow. Patricia Smith of the University of Pennsylvania Press provided valuable and much appreciated editorial assistance and friendly, caring support throughout the preparation of the manuscript.

I am grateful for all the help I received in looking for a visual representation of critical care nursing practice. I received great interest, assistance, and cooperation in searching for and finding the cover photograph. Debra Bloom, Director of Public Relations and Insitutional Advancement, Crawford Long Hospital, Atlanta, Georgia; Ann Borden, Director of University Photography, Emory University, Atlanta, Georgia; Lee Jenkins, Publication Media Director, Emory University Hospital; Karen Schindler, Director of Publications, Woodruff Health Science Center, Emory University; and Jeanine Jackson, RN, MN, CNNP, all contributed to this effort. Walter Bullington, Al Lundy, Jean Ortiz Pruitt, and Ebba Savage also helped with the search for an appropriate photograph. I thank them all.

I particularly thank the very special nurses with whom I take care of patients at Emory University Hospital.

I have felt very supported and cared for by my family and friends throughout this effort. I thank them, heartily.

Finally, I am grateful to the critical care nurses who spoke so openly to me about their experiences with patients. I have been touched and enriched by them. Because of the sensitive nature of the interview material, I am unable to thank them by name.

Introduction

Critical care nursing is the nursing of people undergoing life-threatening physiological crises. According to the American Association of Critical Care Nurses (AACN), "the scope of critical care nursing is defined by the dynamic interaction of the critically ill patient, the critical care nurse and the critical care environment" (American Association of Critical Care Nurses, 1984). Critical care nursing may be distinguished from nursing practice in general by the severity of the patient's illness, the particular skills of the nurse, and the setting where the nursing is practiced. Joan Lynaugh and Julie Fairman distinguish two criteria inherent in the meaning of critical care. "First, the person receiving care is physiologically unstable and at risk of dying. Second, intensive care is usually given in the expectation or hope, however slim, of the person's survival. The relationship between them [these criteria] changes over time" (Lynaugh and Fairman, 1992: 20).

Critical care units emerged in American hospitals after World War II. Medical specialization, increasingly sophisticated medical technology, and advances in anesthesia, cardiology, and surgery influenced this phenomenon. Nathan Simon attributes the development of the modern intensive care unit (ICU) concept to three major forces. First, the recovery room experience in the 1940s and 1950s demonstrated to medicine and nursing the effectiveness of continuous nursing surveillance of very ill patients. Patients waking up after anesthesia and surgery could be monitored in one large room for immediate complications such as respiratory distress, cardiac or blood pressure abnormalities, or bleeding. Second, hospital planners proposed a progressive patient care concept: patients in hospitals would be grouped according to the amount and intensity of nursing care required. Their goal was efficiency—the best matching of nurses with patients. Third, complex technology, medical specialization, and new surgical procedures required more sophisticated postoperative nursing care (Simon, 1980: 2–3). The development in the early 1960s of cardiopulmonary resuscitation (CPR) machines for monitoring heart rhythm (cardiac monitors) and DC (direct current) defibrillation for the treatment of lethal arrhythmias after heart attacks ushered in the era of the coronary care unit (Hilberman, 1975: 162).

The Joint Commission on Accreditation of Healthcare Organizations (JCAHO) defines a special care unit as one "that provides intensive care continuously on a 24-hour-a-day basis. Specific purpose special care units may include, but need not be limited to burn, cardiac, cardiovascular surgery, neonatal, respiratory units, and multipurpose special care units that usually include medical-surgical intensive care units or a combination of the above" (*AMH 92*, 1992: 157). American Hospital Association records indicate that, in 1979, one in fifteen U.S. hospital beds was designated for critically ill patients (Disch, 1981: 1050). The majority of all hospitals (61%) have one specific critical care unit providing combined medical-surgical care. Medical centers or university teaching hospitals are likely to have more than one unit, each providing specialty care — for example, heart surgery, neurosurgery, organ transplant (liver, pancreas, kidney, heart, heart-lung, or bone marrow), pulmonary, or trauma units (Kinney, 1981: 1051). Hence, intensive care is now a usual standard of care in U.S. hospitals. Patients may be admitted to an intensive care unit for an acute illness like pneumonia or a heart attack; for short-term management after specialized surgery such as coronary artery bypass surgery; or for long-term management of complications of either — for example, a patient on a ventilator for respiratory support after respiratory arrest during treatment for pneumonia.

U.S. hospitals in the 1990s face an on-going crisis brought about by economic, political, and social conditions in the larger society. First, the medical care establishment in the United States has been illness-oriented, and both the insurance industry and federal health care programs have supported this priority. Some shifts toward prevention, health maintenance programs, and ambulatory care have occurred, but these efforts remain in the minority. Hospital care is expensive, and because of federal funding cuts, increasing numbers of Americans, especially the poor, have no access to medical care (Freeman et al., 1987).

Second, the population characteristics of hospital patients are changing. Patients are older, with more complex health problems, and are sicker at every age when they arrive at a hospital for care (Freeman et al., 1987). Prospective payment or managed care systems imposed by insurers, including Medicare, reduce the length of hospital stays. Consequently, patients are discharged earlier with more illness needs and less independence than ever before. The spread of acquired immune deficiency syndrome (AIDS) and other communicable diseases like hepatitis and drug-resistant tuberculosis have revolutionized the interpersonal and physical health care environments in all settings.

Third, hospitals in all areas of the United States are increasingly called on to provide comprehensive services, including those requiring highly specialized and technical equipment that may become obsolete very rapidly. These trends are expensive and require large numbers of highly competent personnel, particularly nurses (Garlo, 1984).

Fourth, a nursing shortage of unprecedented proportions is being felt throughout the world, but especially in the United States. The shortage is a result of an increased demand for nurses, a diminishing supply, and an attrition of working nurses from the profession (Georgia Nurses' Association, 1988). Many reasons have been proposed for this shortage: declining numbers of college-aged young people; expanding career opportunities for women; fewer women attracted to nursing; increasing numbers of nurses leaving the field for other careers; nursing's being perceived as low in status, income potential, and employment benefits; the realities of unattractive work schedules; and the risks of hospital environments. On the other hand, current economic conditions and rising unemployment of both men and women in many other occupations have made nursing increasingly attractive. Applications to nursing schools have increased in the past few years, and enrollments are up. Characteristics of graduate nurses and their career paths in the future may be more and more diverse and interesting.

Finally, hospitals have lost nurses to newer settings. Nurses who traditionally worked in hospitals have been attracted to the benefits of home health care and out-patient clinics (Tregarthen, 1987). Changes in Medicare reimbursement to hospitals, introduced in 1983, have encouraged physicians to discharge patients earlier from hospitals. Much of traditional illness care has shifted from hospitals to home and clinic settings. Nurses have left hospitals to work in these environments.

Linda Aiken disputes the premise that the nursing shortage reflects declining numbers. She points out that although actual enrollments in nursing schools have declined some 25 percent since 1984, the numbers of graduates exceeds the numbers of nurses retiring, thus reflecting an increase in the size of the actual pool of nurses. Further, 80 percent of nurses are employed in nursing, a high percentage for a predominantly female occupation (Aiken, 1990: 74–77). The high turnover in hospital nursing positions, Aiken believes, reflects widespread dissatisfaction among nurses with hospital employment. However, since most nurses who resign hospital positions take a job in another hospital, nurse resignations and hospital vacancy rates do not reflect an actual nursing shortage.

Any discussion of nursing practice in critical care requires an introduction to the setting, to the needs of the patient, and to the role of the nurse. The following case study may accomplish this introduction.

NICK: A CASE STUDY

Nick, age 17, was admitted to the hospital intensive care unit (ICU) two days ago. He had rolled his jeep and was thrown from the vehicle, sustaining multiple internal injuries and a head injury. On admission to the hospital, he was taken to surgery for treatment of massive internal bleeding and repair of torn organs. After surgery, Nick was admitted to the ICU for supportive therapy and monitoring. Due to a depressed level of consciousness related to the head injury, he was not breathing sufficiently on his own and required artificial ventilation.

That particular night, the eight-bed ICU was full and four staff nurses were on duty. Nick's nurse had cared for him on the night shift since his admission. Knowing his status well, she was aware of two likely complications: "fluid shifts" resulting in possible hypotension [low blood pressure], and "shock lung" [respiratory distress syndrome]. Nick's last two sets of arterial blood gases (ABGs) [measures of oxygen, carbon dioxide, and pH levels in the arterial blood] showed a dropping blood oxygen content indicating a need to change the settings on the mechanical ventilator to deliver a higher concentration of oxygen.

The doctors had inserted a femoral arterial line which is a fluid filled tube similar to an intravenous (I.V.) line. This line was connected by a pressure transducer to the bedside monitor, allowing for a continuous blood pressure (BP) reading. The monitor and last few recorded vital signs showed Nick's BP to be dropping. Noting the monitor to read 90/60, threateningly low for Nick's condition, his nurse checked the line for accuracy. Finding it was correct, she increased the fluid rate in one of his I.V. lines in an attempt to elevate his BP.

While monitoring the situation, Nick's nurse observed an abnormal heartbeat on the electrocardiograph [EKG] monitor oscilloscope. Watching, she noted more than six of them in a minute, a condition triggering the standard protocol to administer an injection of lidocaine and begin a continuous lidocaine I.V. drip infusion without first obtaining a doctor's order. She left the bedside to prepare the drugs after obtaining an EKG strip to document the arrhythmia.

From the drug preparation area, Nick's nurse continued to watch the monitor. She noted the abnormal beats coming more quickly and sometimes in pairs. Suddenly one abnormal beat occurred during the vulnerable electrical period of a previous normal beat. Nick's heart went into sustained ventricular fibrillation, a life-threatening event.

Nick's nurse called out, "Arrest in four. We've got V-Fib." Gathering the lidocaine and I.V., she rushed to the prepared resuscitation cart containing the defibrillator and pushed it into the room. She plugged in the defibrillator, set it to the appropriate voltage, and applied conducting gel to the paddles. Two other nurses appeared. Nurse A disconnected Nick from the ventilator and began to administer 100 percent oxygen to him by hand using a special bag. At the same time she checked for carotid and femoral pulses, and feeling none announced that fact. Nurse B obtained the board from the cart and together the two positioned it under Nick. Having telephoned the cardiac arrest team and doctor-on-call in the emergency room (ER), Nurse C positioned himself in the central nurses' station to watch all the patient monitors.

Nick's nurse checked the clock. Thirty seconds had elapsed since the "run" of ventricular fibrillation began. "Stand back," she announced, and applying the paddles to Nick's chest, discharged the electrical current. The monitor showed a return to normal sinus heart rhythm. Nurse A administered more oxygen by hand, and then reconnected Nick to the ventilator, adjusting its settings to provide larger volumes and more oxygen. Nick's nurse administered the lidocaine and set up the I.V. drip utilizing a mechanical infusion pump to deliver precisely four milligrams per minute. Nick's condition had been stabilized.

Nick's nurse made a quick check on the patient in the next room. The second patient under her care was a 45-year-old alcoholic woman admitted with severe, but now controlled, gastrointestinal bleeding. She still required a close watch, however, due to the potential for rebleeding and delirium tremens. The nurse noted her to be restless and disoriented, but luckily restrained so as to prevent self-harm. Returning to Nick's room, his nurse began to chart the recent events.

The cardiac arrest team never arrived because it had already responded to an emergency in another part of the hospital. The ER doctor finally arrived and brought news of a drug overdose patient in the ER who needs an ICU bed. The time is 2:30 a.m. and the nurses must prepare to transfer their "least sick" patient. (Garlo, 1984: 240–242)

While this case study may sound dramatic, it illustrates many features of critical care nursing practice. The practicing nurse in critical care settings is a participant in the most intimate life and death events that persons can experience in dealing with illness. Other medical groups share this domain with nursing. Physicians, clergy, physical and respiratory therapists, social workers, and hospital administrators are among the many professionals who interact with critically ill patients and their families in the modern hospital. But the characteristics of nursing practice in hospitals make the role of the nurse unique among the various professional groups that serve patients and their families. The particular skills, the persistence of caring, and the continuous round-the-clock presence of nurses in hospitals form a triad that renders nursing distinctive from other health groups.

Nurses may assume a special role with very ill patients in which direct and continuous support of physiological, emotional, social, and spiritual functions is provided.

Nurses may use a wide variety of skills and techniques to take care of patients. A problem-solving or nursing process approach is generally accepted by professional and educational groups; practice, licensing, and accrediting bodies; and the institutions where nursing is practiced as an appropriate framework for nursing practice and activities (ANA, 1980; *AMH 87*, 1987; *AMH 92*, 1992; Holloway, 1993; Hudak, Gallo, and Lohr, 1990; Kinney, Packa, and Dunbar, 1993; Moorhouse, Geissler, and Doenges, 1987). This approach includes assessing and diagnosing patient problems, planning and goal setting for individual patient needs, intervening for each problem, and evaluating results. Pain and anxiety are examples of patient problems for which nurses might intervene. In hospitals, nurses might be involved in direct care of patients, management, teaching, research, or consultation regarding patient care. Nursing roles in hospitals may also encompass coordinating the multiple services involved in patient care.

The direct care nursing role in critical care settings involves assessing the complex interplay of illness or dysfunction of the individual as a physiologic and psychologic whole. The nurse may be considered an extension of the functions of a person unable to care for him- or herself. The patient crisis may be elective surgery, overwhelming infection, trauma, angina, or multiple system failure and coma. The nurse provides physical care and monitors vital functions including heart rate; blood pressure; skin integrity; bowel and bladder functions; nutritional, fluid, electrolyte, and mobility status; and mentation. The nurse assesses for abnormalities and takes action to help the patient return to normal function. For example, a nurse may increase intravenous fluids if a postoperative patient seems volume depleted, as evidenced by low urine output, rapid heart rate, low blood pressure, and poor skin turgor. On the other hand, a nurse may discontinue oral fluids or food in this same patient in the presence of abdominal distension and decreased bowel sounds. Critical care nurses, using parameters and "judgments" related to interacting factors, routinely titrate drip rates of very potent drugs that affect the heart, blood pressure, cardiac output, and blood sugar level. The special skills and experiences that the nurse possesses regarding normal responses to the intrusion of illness provide a basis for judgment. Nursing judgment is difficult to define or quantify, but remains a core competency for any effective nurse in an acute care setting, especially a critical care nurse.

The direct care role makes the nurse a "patient extender." If the patient is paralyzed, the nurse turns the patient to prevent pneumonia and puts all limbs through a passive range of motion to prevent contracture and muscle wasting. If the patient is blind, the nurse will describe the environment of the room so the patient can walk safely. The nursing role goes beyond direct care and involves managing individual responses to illness, rehabilitation, or dying. The nurse may assist the patient and family to assess self-care motivation and potential, to acquire or develop special skills or adaptive equipment, and to obtain reimbursement for acute and long-term care.

In the intensive care unit the nurse collects and monitors vast amounts of detailed data. This monitoring is continuous and occurs in rapidly changing situations. These judgments require anticipation of subtle changes and decision making, interpretations, intervention, and evaluation in complex situations. The outcomes of these decisions may have life and death potential for patients. The decision making may occur in units that are inadequately staffed, organized, and managed and have little or no competent medical back-up. Further, the invasive and life-extending procedures that patients may experience may be perceived as dehumanizing by the nurse and others. When realistic expectation of recovery is lost and the patient's deterioration prolonged, nurses may experience extreme stress at the loss of hope. One nurse expressed the pain of "taking care of dead people. I just can't do it anymore."

The illnesses that place patients in critical care settings are crisis events, often sudden, painful, and excruciating in their impact on patient and family. For example, the crisis of head injury after an automobile accident may be complicated by pregnancy, old age, chronic illness, or AIDS. Decision making by the patient and family is required during a period of high stress, limited knowledge, and consequent dependence on the judgment of medical and nursing personnel. The diagnostic and treatment regimes offered to patients are often ambiguous, and the outcomes may be painful, expensive, and disfiguring. Patients often experience a cycle of incremental decision making, ambiguity, and ambivalence. They encounter machines, procedures, and technology that seem like experimentation or science fiction. They may sense a climate of chaotic unreality, over which they feel no control. The endurance and the outcomes of such experiences are highly stressful for patients and family members. No wonder patients are highly susceptible to stress-related illness such as stress ulcers and psychoses in critical care settings.

The critical care setting has also been shown to be very stressful for hospital staff, and the rate of burnout for physicians and nurses is very high in these areas. Joan L. Stehle (1981), Menzies (1960), and Holsclaw (1965) have noted that nursing in general is seen as stressful because of patient suffering and death, heavy demands, frightening tasks, and disturbing relationships with patients. Nurses feel impotent, especially when they are unable to restore patients to well-being. Although critical care settings have been persistently identified as stressful, Friedman (1982) and Strauss (1968) have noted that factors identified as stressors for some ICU nurses are identified as sources of satisfaction, challenge, and increased staff intimacy and morale by others. Koumans (1965) and Strauss (1968) have identified the following particular stressors for nurses in critical care settings: rapid turnover of staff, intensity of emotions in interpersonal situations, complicated machinery, narrow patient care focus, great responsibility, conflict with administration, and crisis atmosphere. The great variability among these factors indicates the complexity of the critical care setting for nurses, patients, and others. Interestingly, these observations were made in the 1960s, before the rapid increase in technology and specialization.

Altruism and caretaking have been persistent themes throughout the history of nursing (Kalisch and Kalisch, 1986; Melosh, 1982; Reverby, 1987). The roots of nursing altruism have been traced to nineteenth-century reform movements, religion, and traditional women's roles. Susan Reverby has explored the "central dilemma of American nursing: the order to care in a society that refuses to value caring" (Reverby, 1987: 5); her thesis maintains that the order to care was rooted in the duty ascribed to feminine roles. This duty carried obligations but not rights. Nursing therefore must forge a link between altruism and autonomy in order to have "caring-with-autonomy" and "a way of life that includes serving others without being subservient" (Reverby, 1987: 5). Nursing professionalism, the economics of nursing as a predominantly female occupation, the history of both the proposed and actual educational requirements for entry into nursing practice, and the work settings where nursing is practiced are a few of the issues that are influenced by the altruistic roots of nursing. Little attention has been given by scholars to the influence of these issues on the motivation, self-concept, and career choices of nurses and the ways in which various nurses relate to medicine, the hospital, and the larger society.

Contemporary critical care settings engender great potential for loss of human integrity, self-worth, and self-control for patients, family members, and nurses. There is also great potential for meaningful human interaction and intimacy. The nurse is in a position to assist the patient and family to humanize that environment and crisis situation, and perhaps gain some control over life, illness, or death in the hostile hospital environment and create the sort of climate that families and friends might forge in a home setting for an ill loved one.

The central features of the contemporary critical care setting include constant nursing care of complicated patients in highly technical, increasingly specialized, rapidly changing, and complex environments. The moral, social, and ethical dimensions of decision making in these environments are not clear, and the nurse is bound through interpersonal and professional role functions in a pivotal relationship with patient, family, physician, and hospital. Scholars are only beginning to explore the characteristics and dimensions of the stresses and perhaps the satisfactions of these relationships. How distinctive critical care nursing is as a specialty and how representative it is of the discipline as a whole remain questions to be tested relative to traditional roles and to changes affecting nursing and contemporary practice.

Nursing as a discipline and nurses as individuals remain obscure in written histories. Hilberman (1975) documents a chronological history of critical care units with only a passing mention of nurses. Starr (1982) traces the history of the health industry in the United States with only an incidental reference to nursing, the largest group of health care workers in the country. Dorothy Marlow's pediatric nursing textbook (1977: 3–21) gives a history of child care with a list of dates and events of importance, without listing any nursing event or primary sources. Interestingly, by the sixth edition in 1988, the role of the nurse is discussed throughout the section (Marlow and Redding, 1988: 2–16). Nursing is presumed to exist in the shadow of political events and medical accomplishments.

Traditional nursing and medical histories demonstrate class, racial, and sexist biases and problems with primary source materials in addition to their regional biases and their neglect of nursing as an occupation of significance. The documented histories are chronologies of the activities of middle- and upper-class white women, most often told from the perspective of institutional or medical priorities. The primary source materials available pertaining to nursing — for example, the written documentation of nursing school curricula, records of professional nursing organizations, and records of medical treatment — do not reflect the essence of nursing practice. The life experiences and personal commitments of individual nurses remain as obscure as the dimensions of their interactions with patients. Even medical and nursing histories that use primary source materials and portray the unique experience of individuals and minorities are often biased to region. Harris (1978), Kalisch and Kalisch (1986), Melosh (1982), and Reverby (1987) demonstrate a bias toward the northeastern United States in their histories; information about the South, the Midwest, and the West is almost completely absent.

The history of nursing specialty organizations have also remained obscure. In 1988, however, the American Association of Critical Care Nurses awarded a grant to conduct research for the purpose of writing a history of the organization. Lynaugh and Fairman (1992) have provided a preview of their research on AACN's history conducted at the Center for the Study of the History of Nursing at the University of Pennsylvania and report that a book on the full history will be forthcoming.

As G. Grob notes, social history approaches to the history of disease and medicine can reveal fundamental values in American society "and reflect the size and structure of the population, the social structure, technology, and living and cultural pattern in society" (Grob, 1977: 396). In recent years social historians and others have reduced many of the kinds of biases that have been discussed above. Further, they have begun to ask more appropriate questions and to acknowledge the limitations of existing data. This trend has been furthered by interests in the nurse as worker, as female, as hospital employee, and as participant in grassroots health care. Still, the practicing nurse is less visible in written histories than the bureaucratic education and practice organizations.

As an occupational history of a largely female group, the story of the evolution of nursing, particularly critical care nursing, provides a view of changing women's roles since World War II. It also provides a perspective on the ways in which nurses and nursing have interacted with individuals, other occupations, and institutions — notably, patients, medicine, and hospitals respectively. Nursing has been the persistent human factor in the evolution of critical care units in U.S. hospitals. Nurses are the largest group of workers in hospitals and are the only hospital employees with consistent, round-the-clock contact with patients. Hence, the history of critical care nursing reflects the many changes in hospital care of patients that have occurred since World War II. Most visible among these changes have been the emergence of medical specialization and the increased use of highly technical equipment for diagnosis, treatment, and direct patient care at the bedside.

A study of the characteristics of nursing practice in ICU settings reveals information about the ways in which nurses, patients, and others respond to the complex, stressful, and highly technical critical care environment. A study of critical care nursing is also a valuable source of information about the interactions between nurses and patients and their families, physicians, and others; the actual nursing care delivered; and the ethical dimensions of critical care practice.

The structure and organization of contemporary critical care units are predictable and reflect external standards and regulations. The nursing literature reflects a young, self-absorbed discipline largely concerned with professional standards, education, leadership, and performance issues. The human, interpersonal experience of nursing practice and the knowledge inherent in practice have received less attention.

Dolores Garlo studied the legal dimensions of the evolution of critical care nursing, and proposed that the application of technology resulted in the critical care nursing specialty. The distinctiveness of critical care nursing and its representation of nursing as a general discipline await description. Certainly the nurse, the patient, and a high concentration of technology and equipment define the critical care setting. R. Vreeland and G. L. Ellis (1969) have made a significant observation about the paradoxical nature of the ICU nurse's situation, where warmth and sympathy are expected together with objectivity and assertiveness.

My motivation for studying the history of critical care nursing practice is rooted in three distinct but merging realities. First, my experience since the mid-1960s as a hospital nurse and nursing educator in Pennsylvania, Florida, and Georgia has coincided with the development of critical care nursing. I have been a critical care nurse in two community hospitals and a teaching hospital and have taught associate, baccalaureate, and master of nursing students in critical care, and I have lived with the increasing complexity in these settings. I have been amazed at the ability of nurses, and I include myself, to take on responsibility for so much technical equipment and continue to be available for both the human needs of patients and their families and the traditional nursing concerns of patient teaching, physical and emotional caregiving, and supervising the activities of daily living. It seems that nurses do everything and are constantly taking on more. The challenges to accomplish "everything" are hypnotic, and the costs are insidious. Stress effects, mechanistic performance or even incompetence, and "burnout" are a few of the very real outcomes. Also very real and powerful are the intimacies between nurses and patients and/or their families in these highly stressful settings. An energy potential, almost like a stretched rubber band, can permeate these interactions.

I know that nurses make a difference to patients and families and to their own humanity when they intervene in the debilitating, dehumanizing, and ethically demanding situations that can occur as a consequence of "high-tech" treatment. I have seen nurses take control of the details of these settings and empower hopelessly ill or dying patients and their families to make choices and get some control and humanity back into their lives. Other persons, especially physicians and chaplains, are involved, but nurses are with patients constantly. I know that these interactions with patients are intimate and powerful and at the core of the skills, attitudes, and values that define nursing practice: competence, caring, and commitment. That story of nursing is not reported in any of the literature of nursing or other disciplines.

My interest in social history, especially women's history, since nursing has been so predominantly female, precipitated the second reality. The traditional histories I looked at did not reflect the human experience of caretaking, both because of the narrow selection of sources and because of the priorities of the writers. Traditional nursing histories did not reflect the intimacy of my experiences.

The third reality occurred when I was introduced to the outcomes of oral history methods while studying the Nazi Holocaust. Listening to the experiences of concentration camp survivors and the military liberators of the camps, I soon realized the potential in oral history to capture the "heart" of human experience.

Oral tradition has been viewed as an acceptable substitute for the written record, as an art form representative of a particular culture and time, and as a unique expression of human dimensions not readily found in written records (Abzug, 1985; Bellah et al., 1985; Hall, Korstad, and Leloudis, 1986). R. H. Abzug describes the impact of oral interviews with American liberators of the concentration camps: "they afford us a window on the way men and women act and think when faced with the unimaginable suffering of others. The deep compassion and sometimes the limits of vision displayed . . . pointed to important ambivalences about facing the Holocaust and its victims . . . and the immediate and long-range impact of their discoveries on the public mind" (Abzug, 1985: x). It is this latter characteristic that makes oral interviews an appropriate method for examining the experiences of critical care nurses. Written records, excepting autobiographies, if they exist, are an inadequate reflection of the quality of nurses' experiences with human suffering and human potential.

The purpose of this study is to explore the evolution and contemporary practice of critical care nursing from the perspective of the practicing nurse through the use of oral history methods. The following questions will be explored:

- What has been the experience of nurses in critical care units during a period of increasing specialization and the use of rapidly changing and complex technology?
- What is the essence of nursing practice in critical care settings?
- What are the practice issues and the range of nurses' responses to the ethical dimensions of critical care nursing practice?

I conducted extensive interviews with twenty-five nurses who represented a range of critical care experience. Participants were selected to represent: experience in critical care settings from the 1950s to the present; work in rural and urban areas, in teaching and private hospitals, in Veteran's Administration (VA) and non-military hospitals; diversity in age, sex, race, and educational background; and a range of staff, management, and clinical experiences in hospitals. A detailed description and critique of the methodology, the forms developed for the study, and sample characteristics are included in the Appendix. Conducted over a one-year period from March 1987 to March 1988, the interviews were taped and lasted from one to two hours. Interviews were held in my home, in nurses' homes, and in private offices in hospital or nursing school settings, as determined by the convenience for the nurse as well as considerations of privacy and tape quality.

The nurses very openly discussed their experiences, impressions, and beliefs about critical care nursing. Many of them described intimate experiences with critically ill and dying patients that matched my own. Further, I had the impression that for many of these nurses, as for me, this research provided their first opportunity to speak so openly and in such detail about the meaning of nursing in their lives. They discussed stressful and interpersonal factors in the setting that were constraints and enhancers and described their necessary but often difficult relationships with medicine and with the hospital administration. Finally, the nurses identified and described the stresses, ethical issues, and patient needs they confronted in practice and identified the nursing measures they used to care for patients.

The first chapter examines the evolution of the concept of critical care and the realities of the intensive care unit (ICU) and coronary care unit (CCU) that developed, and explores the characteristics of the critical care setting and the realities of the practice of nursing that emerged: first, the effects of technology on the setting and personnel; second, the specific impact of medical specialization on the role of the critical care nurse; third, nursing practice in the context of the technology and environment; fourth, the new role of the nurse in the CCU and surgical ICU. The chapter concludes with a discussion of contemporary issues that influence critical care practice, especially the current shortage of nurses in the United States.

Chapter 2 presents the voices of critical care nurses illustrating the history and practice issues presented in Chapter 1. The nurses talk about the evolution of the intensive care unit and the coronary care unit and the multiple effects of technology on patient care and nursing practice. Two excerpts from interviews with Edith Hardeman and Karen Adler provide a sampling of the value of these experiences. Edith Hardeman is a 38-year-old nurse with 17 years of nursing experience, 1970, in South Carolina, North Carolina, Alabama, and Georgia. Most of those years have been spent in medical cardiology both in community hospitals and in medical center teaching hospitals. Hardeman describes her experiences through the years as cardiology has changed from passive support of patients having heart attacks to highly technical and sophisticated diagnostic and intervention measures such as cardiac catheterization, balloon angioplasty, open heart surgery, and drugs to protect the heart and prevent or treat damaged muscle:

The one thing that bothered me more than any other, as I started going along in cardiology, was the fact that we would see the same patients over and over again. Every time they came in they had knocked off another chunk of their myocardium and we weren't really doing anything to prevent it. A doctor in Alabama used to tell his patients when they had their infarct [heart attack], "Well, you know all that pain that you have been having, now that this is about ready to happen, you aren't going to have it any more." Of course, they didn't have any left ventricle any more. We just didn't do a lot to prevent it.

I remember the first patient I ever took care of was an MI [a patient with a myocardial infarction, a heart attack], when I was in nursing school before we had the CCU. We kept him in bed for six weeks and then we kept him on "bed to chair" for six weeks and the only monitoring he got was the pulse rate we were taking at the radius [wrist], and we gave him Coumadin [to prevent blood clots] because we kept him in bed long enough to have clots. He could have been one big clot from head to toe. I saw that care progress and that felt good because we were getting into cardiac rehabilitation. But you still had the feeling that it was a progressive disease and you were watching them decline. Every time they came in they were a little bit worse.

As I am at a medical center now and we are doing PTCAs [percutaneous transluminal coronary angioplasty, or balloon angioplasty] and we've done a tPA [tissue plasminogen, an activator drug that dissolves clots in coronary arteries] study and we're actively intervening. The nurse who used to look at twelve lead electrocardiograms for localization of infarct as an exercise, is now looking at the EKG and calling up the physician, as I have on many occasions, and saying: "Your patient is showing signs of an acute inferior infarct now. We need to take him somewhere now and do something now." And having it done and realizing that you are very instrumental in keeping an infarct down or the size down or giving them a chance anyway.

I find what we do is a mixed blessing. I certainly find that some of the patients would have died a long time ago if we had not taken care of them for months and months. Their cardiomyopathy [diseased heart] isn't ever going to get any better and we are trying to save them. I find that frustrating. To a certain extent, we still see them come back, just pulling off a chunk of muscle every time.

Hardeman's reflections demonstrate the impact of technology on enlarging treatment methods, the changed roles of physicians and nurses, and the complex environments in which care takes place. Further, it demonstrates the ambiguities of treatment. Intervention prolongs life but does not cure the disease process. Ethical dimensions of treatment and quality of life issues are inherent in this scenario.

Karen Adler, 35 years old, who has experiences in rehabilitation and two medical-surgical intensive care units over ten years, beginning in 1977, describes the stresses of critical care:

Nurses work in situations that other professionals would not even begin to put up with. We do. We tend to work in rather difficult situations a lot of times, not only with the emotional load that we are carrying but just the physical stress of the situation. Taking care of somebody who is trying their damndest to die and you are trying your damndest to keep them alive for an intense twelve-hour period of time where you don't have a break, where you are having to deal with multiple people back and forth and you get very few pats on the back from anybody. That to me is the real basis of burnout. You turn around and you look and say, "I just can't do this any more for one reason or another." Then you move on to another job, another position.

You job-hop for a while or you get to a point where you can finally decide what things you can accept and what things you are going to ignore. I think that it is the stress that does in critical care nurses, and I have seen a lot of our nurses leave because the death rate on our unit is just so phenomenal. It is just so hard to be giving 100 percent all of the time, knowing that very few of them are going to make it out of that situation. After awhile you just start asking yourself, "Why even bother?"

The interviews with Edith Hardeman and Karen Adler reflect a progression in the nurse's role toward increasing medical specialization and enlarged treatment methods, as well as the stresses of the care and the setting.

Chapter 3 deals with the intimacy of the nurse-patient interaction. Nurses describe their motivations, satisfaction, and frustration with nursing care. The stresses of care are especially dealt with. Emily Vereen is an experienced forty-two-year-old nurse who has worked for twenty-four years, beginning in 1964, with critically ill cancer patients. Her description of her day with a Mrs. A reveals much about the creativity and sensitivity that can come with maturity and experience in clinical nursing practice:

Mrs. A is a patient that the staff decided was a pain in the butt. I said that I would take her. I walked into the room and everything hurt. So I kind of sized her up real quickly and tried not to take into account anything that I heard about her, so I said, "Me too." Everything that she said I said, "Me too. That's the way I'm feeling too, Mrs. A." She said, "I am complaining a whole hellava lot, aren't I?" I said, "Yes." She said, "Are you my nurse for the day?" I said, "Yes, but you did not even allow me the time to tell you that. You made me your priest, your rabbi. But I am going to be all of that today. Anything that you need me to be I am going to be and you are going to be mine because I need some TLC today too. So we are going to do it for each other."

That was unorthodox, but it worked for her. She was able to get up for the first time in seven days, and we got a bath, we washed her hair, we had lipstick on, and we had a brand new lady by the end of the day. There was something about her personality that I could perceive that she would respond to me. I did not go too far so that I could not correct it if she did not respond to me in the right way. There is something about intuitive balance that you can't teach and I thought, "Well, an instructor might not ever do this, but it worked."

She is up. She requested no pain medicine. She yelled at nobody. She was not unreasonable. All she needed was to be loved. She had nobody here, no visitors. All she needed was to be cared about.

Unorthodox management sometimes works for unorthodox situations and you have to know to try whatever it takes to help that person cope. Dying is something that we think about sometimes, but just sit down and think about it today. The doctor comes and says, "There is nothing else that I can do for you." You are lying there and your door is closed and everybody else walks by. Nobody wants to come see you and you are wondering, "When is death coming?" By the middle of the afternoon you know what her question was? "Do you think that I am going to die tomorrow or the next day?" Can you imagine the agony that she lived? Nobody wants to die tomorrow unless you have accepted that as inevitable. You are not ready to die tomorrow, unless you are ready to die tomorrow. We have to know how to help in those kinds of situations.

Vereen's story of her interaction with Mrs. A reveals much about sensitive listening, caring, and effective intervention. Chapter 3 presents interviews with other nurses who describe many other satisfactions about nursing care and the many stresses that operate in these settings. Of particular note are stresses that interfere with delivering the quality of care that Mrs. A received from Emily Vereen.

Chapter 4 considers the ethical issues that the critical care nurses interviewed identified as most significant to their practice: death with dignity for hopelessly ill patients who may experience radical forms of treatment, withdrawal of life-support measures, or "do not resuscitate" designation; issues surrounding organ transplant; and quality of life issues related to resource allocation and decision making. The meaning of language and the impact of such factors as age, AIDS, and costly, experimental treatment on quality of life issues are identified by nurses as introducing significant ethical dimensions to patient care in critical care settings.

Denise Clements, 39, with twelve years of critical care experience in five hospitals in a metropolitan southern city, beginning in 1975, is now a clinical manager in a surgical intensive care unit in a teaching hospital. She speaks about the ethical issues that affect her staff:

We're seeing sicker patients than I've ever seen in my life and I've been doing this for quite a while. We are keeping people alive that we would have let go long before. Multiple interventions—with higher complexity—that feel a little like experimentation. We're doing painful things and prolonging suffering in the elderly or in people who really are not going to be able to have much quality to their lives. And the AIDS epidemic. Those are the things that are getting to the staff more than anything else.

Is it ethical to take a patient to surgery and other invasive procedures when you know that patient is going to be dead within a matter of days? That happened last week. And the woman was in advanced age. She had sarcoidosis and was infected and bleeding, and they were doing all these procedures on her. And we were just insane over it. Is it ethical to fill up coronary care units with people needing heart transplants and maybe not have enough resources to take care of someone who's got a treatable heart attack—a 48-year-old who could really benefit from your coronary care unit? But—no beds, because you're holding all of them for people who should be dead. We're trying to keep them alive so we can try this odd thing. Is it ethical to not restrain a patient who is intubated on a ventilator, who has AIDS, knowing that the patient is going to pull his own endotracheal tube or ventilator to commit suicide? And that happened to us. Are we going to look the other way and let you commit suicide, but not go ahead and give you morphine and end your life in a more humane manner? I've even seen the opposite of that where it has seemed very unethical to me to deny morphine to an AIDS patient who refused intubation and was gasping for breath and whose anxiety was—he was in the final moments before death and we couldn't give him anything to ease the discomfort in those moments because the physician said, and I quote, "We don't want to sedate him." You know, things like that where nurses are crying and saying, "I don't need this. I don't have to feel this."

Clements presents many of the ethical issues that critical care nurses confront daily. Chapter 4 describes nurses' perceptions about these and other dilemmas, especially problems related to extraordinary treatment. Nurses also describe strategies that they use to cope with these stresses.

Chapter 5 brings together the several unifying themes that emerged from the interviews with critical care nurses. The critical care unit has become increasingly complex and highly technical. Nurses have rapidly become the major treatment modality in the critical care unit because of skill, competence in judgment, and round-the-clock presence. These skills are additive. Nurses incorporate them into the traditional caring role, and they are a source of satisfaction and stress. The commitment of the critical care nurse to patients and to nursing practice is passionate and personal. Nurses believe that they make a difference to patients through competence, advocacy, and coordination and management of the clinical environment. The ethical dimensions of critical care nursing, especially those related to factors that interfere with death with dignity, are sources of conflict and stress. Critical care nurses express ambivalence and conflict about the necessary but difficult relationships between nursing and both medicine and the hospital as an organization.

The voices of these critical care nurses reflect the values of American society and reveal much about human limitations and human potential. They speak of the ways in which economic and political issues influence health care. Finally, their stories present a case study of an occupation whose unique combination of expert skill, caring, and flexibility may provide a model for society on appropriate ways to manage technology, change, and complexity as the U.S. health care system is reconsidered in the 1990s.

1. The Evolution of Critical Care Nursing

Critical care nursing is a post-World War II phenomenon. Its development paralleled the rise of medical specialization and the rapid emergence of complex medical technology. According to N. M. Simon (1980:2–3), the modern intensive care unit (ICU) concept owes its development to three major forces. First, the recovery room experience in the 1940s and 1950s has shown to medicine and nursing the advantage of intensive and continual surveillance, by nurses, of very ill patients. Second, the progressive patient care concept proposed by hospital planners determined that patients in hospitals would be grouped according to the amount and intensity of nursing care required, in facilities designed to meet their special needs. Third, an evolving complex technology that permitted more ambitious surgical procedures required increasingly complex postoperative surveillance and nursing care.

The direct antecedent of the intensive care unit was the postoperative recovery room, which came into common use in the 1950s. Prerequisite and concurrent developments included those as diverse as antiseptic surgery, X-ray, blood transfusion, the hypodermic needle and syringe, the ventilator, cardiopulmonary resuscitation, various types of anesthesia, and drugs for pain relief, immunization, and antibiotics (Harmer and Henderson, 1955; Kalisch and Kalisch, 1986; Starr, 1982). Treatment of battle casualties during World War II and the Korean and Vietnam wars produced new surgical techniques and treatment and supported the growth of critical care nursing as a specialty. Factors as varied as the role of women in the military and the emergence of the helicopter for triage and evacuation of the wounded for treatment elsewhere further refined the role of the critical care nurse.

The post-World War II trend toward hospital staff employment for nurses coincided with the boom in hospital building precipitated by federal funds for hospital construction (Melosh, 1982). Specialization continued within medicine, paralleling new technologies and developments in cardiac surgery and arteriography, such as the heart-lung machine. Chemotherapeutic drugs and radiation in the treatment of cancer also developed during this period. The emergence of Medicare and Medicaid in the 1960s coincided with the struggle for equal rights for women and minority groups in the United States, and influenced health care availability and access for these groups. The development of oral contraceptives ushered in an era of changed sexual mores and family patterns. These events coincided with concerns about nuclear destruction, the pollution of the environment, and electronic developments such as the transistor and the twentieth-century microchip. The recent emergence of acquired immune deficiency syndrome (AIDS) has presented the threat of a major global epidemic that as yet has no effective treatment or cure. The health care industry, reflecting society, has only begun to confront the enormous implications of this disease.

Developments in nursing education and practice may be examined in the context of the aforementioned rapid social and technological changes, which have had impacts on health and illness. After World War II, federal dollars were increasingly available for nursing education, and nurses were assured employment in increasing numbers of hospitals and various health agencies (Georgia Nurses' Association, 1988). In the 1970s, 1980s, and 1990s, hospitals became more specialized and costly, but simultaneously there was a trend toward health promotion, improved nutrition and exercise, and outpatient care.

Critical care nursing developed during the phase of medical specialization in the 1960s. By 1970, hospitals were the third largest industry in the United States, surpassed only by the steel and automobile industries. The coronary care unit, established in 1962, greatly improved patients' chances of surviving heart attacks, and nurses with specialized knowledge were required to care for these patients. Just as nurses practiced in recovery rooms and specialized surgical intensive care units, the coronary care unit nurses "nursed" in another new setting with refined skills and broadened scopes of practice that perhaps often challenged existing nurse practice acts (Garlo, 1984: 249). As new specialties, including neurosurgery, organ transplantation, burn treatment, and trauma care, developed, specialized intensive care units emerged to care for patients in these units. Nursing was designed to support the physical and psychosocial needs of patients moving through periods of crisis resolution toward recovery, rehabilitation, or death.

The common thread through this trend toward specialization was the practice of expert nursing for twenty-four hours a day, in increasingly complex environments. A specialty organization, the American Association of Critical Care Nurses, emerged in the 1970s. This group published a professional journal, defined critical care practice and education standards, conducted national meetings, provided regional and local workshops and chapter organizations, promoted a certification examination for critical care nurses, and sponsored critical care nursing research.

Critical care nursing cannot be understood in isolation from nursing as a professional discipline. While geographical and specialization designations such as the emergency room, the coronary care unit, the Mobile Army Surgical Hospital (MASH) unit, or the intensive care unit may imply critical care, the distinctiveness of critical care nursing awaits description. In fact, little scholarship exists to indicate whether critical care nursing represents a concentration of nursing practice as a whole or reflects something innovative and different. Further, the impact of specialization and the rapid influx of technological change on nursing practice has gained the attention of few researchers. The uniqueness of nursing practice in these settings has received even less attention.

Similarly, as in nursing in general, little is known about the human dimensions of the practice of a critical care nurse. The critical care nurse lives twenty-four hours a day, seven days a week, in highly stressful, intellectually demanding, and rapidly changing environments, with and for patients with multiple needs. This patient population is sicker and older than before, with more complex health problems requiring a variety of interventions (Freeman et al., 1987). Further, critical care nurses are now at risk of exposure to life-threatening diseases like AIDS, hepatitis, and tuberculosis and injury from toxic products and processes such as x-rays in the environment. The involvement of the nurse with the patient, the patient's family and friends, the physicians, and other health care personnel may exemplify a model of communication and practice that is unique. Little is known about the motivation of critical care nurses for involving themselves in these situations and assuming these risks.

There is, unfortunately, little scholarship on this aspect of nursing practice. Certainly the conflict in values and beliefs and the ethical and moral dimensions of nursing practice in these settings merit further study. Finally, a scholarly caution is in order. The statements above can describe nurse-patient interactions not traditionally described as critical care, by nurses not defined as critical care nurses. The designation of critical care nursing as distinctive and unique, or as representative of the discipline as a whole, remains a question for study. The examination of the development of critical care nursing practice that follows may help illuminate these questions.

The History of Critical Care Nursing

A formal comprehensive history of critical care nursing has not been written. Most discussions of the development of either critical care nursing or the critical care unit have addressed dimensions of three closely associated phenomena: the rapid emergence of a highly technical medical environment, medical and nursing specialization, and the associated changes in hospital organization and personnel. These developments have been relatively recent and change has occurred very rapidly.

The roots of medical technology and specialization have been traced to antiquity. Aristotle (384–322 B.C.) distinguished the arteries from the veins, and Galen (A.D. 129–199) noted that the arteries, when cut, always "gushed blood." He applied a tie, or tourniquet, to arteries to stop bleeding (Kalisch and Kalisch, 1986: 6). If we accept technology as "applied science, a technical method for achieving a practical purpose" (*Webster*, 1988), the use of the tourniquet may represent the application of a new technology in ancient Greece. As J. D. Bolter (1984) points out, tools epitomize the stages of human development; clay pottery, the clock, and the steam engine represent progressive stages of development. To this sequence Bolter adds the computer, predicting that future intellectual efforts will involve the use of computers.

In analyzing technology as a shaping force in contemporary society, I. L. Bennett, Jr. notes that technology is often defined as the practical application of scientific research. Although this assessment is limited, it is true that public concern with problems created by technological change such as the deterioration of family life, alienation, boredom, anxiety, drug use, and mental illness often focuses blame on the scientific community. Further, the scientist may be seen as a culprit by people who fear the nuclear annihilation, pollution, extinction of plant and animal species, and dehumanization that are often associated with technological development.

New technologies may be classified as substitute or add-on technologies. New technology may substitute a better, more efficient way of accomplishing something previously possible or may add on or make possible something previously unknown. Most new medical technologies are add-ons. They accomplish something, at increased cost, that was not previously possible. However, they do not necessarily increase productivity in the health establishment or reduce cost to the consumer or to society. Furthermore, decisions about new medical technologies may be based on the technologies' perceived impact on lessening disability and pain and prolonging life or on access to decision makers about funding priorities (Bennett, 1977: 125–133).

According to Bennett, the medical establishment appears to deviate from adherence to the principle that market demand stimulates technological advances. Several factors seem to be at work in contributing to the reality that Lewis Thomas has described — that "in medicine, it is characteristic of technology that we do not count the cost, ever, even when the bills begin coming in" (in Bennett, 1977: 126). First, the consumer of medical technology is now the physician rather than the patient. It is the physician who orders hospitalization, diagnostic tests, surgery, and drugs. Second, the physician follows the concept of technological imperative — the belief that all physicians, patients, and hospitals should have available all the technologies of medicine, regardless of cost, priorities, or allocation of resources. The supplier creates the demand. Third, the reimbursement system for payment of medical costs historically has been less influenced by market forces than have other parts of the economy. Recent changes in Medicare reimbursement, however, suggest alterations from a system where the physician or hospital creates the demand, sets the cost, and guarantees payment (Bennett, 1977: 126–127).

Many thoughtful individuals in various disciplines have reflected on the meaning of the machine for quality of life issues that influence the interplay of individuals and the larger society and the planet. In his examination of the interplay of technical developments in Western civilization with aspects of the social, scientific, and political milieu, Lewis Mumford (1934) describes the clock as the key machine of the modern age. Once the technical development of the clock was given substance in the ordered monastic tradition "time-keeping passed into time-serving and time-accounting and time-rationing. Time replaced eternity as the measure of human action" (1934: 14).

Alvin Toffler and John Naisbitt (1982) have provided commentaries on the evolutionary and revolutionary changes predicted in the transition from an industrial to an information world. Because of their articulation of issues and their media visibility, both men have had an impact on the larger society and on scholarly and applied work in this area. Toffler (1970, 1980) describes a third new era of human existence, a synthesizing, future-oriented era replacing the agricultural and industrial eras that preceded it. The trend is toward global, open, multi-option, emerging realities. Naisbitt (1982) similarly describes an emerging U.S. society that is being restructured in profoundly technical ways. The U.S. economy is now based more on information than on industrialization. New technology imposes a human response at each phase. Economic considerations are focused more on global and long-term considerations than on national and short-term issues. Centralization, institutional help, representative democracy, and formal hierarchies are being replaced by decentralization, self-help, participatory democracy, and networking. Americans are migrating to the South and West and abandoning the industrial North. Finally, a narrow, either/or society is moving toward a multiple-option society, one in which diversity in lifestyle, economics, and social patterns is possible.

According to Fritzof Capra, society faces a transitional crisis similar to the change in concepts and ideas from the mechanistic views of Descartes and Newton to the more holistic and ecological view that occurred in physics as a result of the exploration of the atomic and sub-atomic world in the early twentieth century. Capra proposes a new paradigm, or vision of reality, that would include the "emerging systems view of life, mind, consciousness, and evolution; the corresponding holistic approach to health and healing. The integration of western and eastern approaches to psychology and psychotherapy; a new conceptual framework for economics and technology; and an ecological and feminist perspective which is spiritual in its ultimate nature and will lead to profound changes in our societal and political structure" (Capra, 1982: 16–17).

J. P. Martino (1993) proposes a decision-making model of technological forecasting in which methodological and statistical techniques are incorporated into a decision-making framework for use by engineers, scientists, and administrators. The significance of this model, in the context of this discussion, is the fact that such a framework is intended to command the realities of present and future technologies.

According to Alfred North Whitehead (1931), the relationship between the time span of major cultural change and the life span of individuals determines the nature of education. As long as the time span of cultural change exceeds the life span of individuals, education can be considered the transmission of knowledge. In essence, what individuals learn in their youth remains valid for the rest of their lives. In the twentieth century, the time span of cultural change is considerably shorter than the human life span. Thus, training and education must prepare individuals to face a variety of conditions. Whitehead's observations have direct application in the area of enlarging medical and nursing technologies.

As A. W. Mathies, Jr. (1978) has described, profound changes in medical education and practice have occurred as a result of emerging life-support technologies. Early attempts in the 1940s to assist premature infants with the new techniques of oxygen administration and the use of the antibiotic chloramphenical resulted in retrolental fibroplasia and gray baby syndrome respectively. These iatrogenic problems actively improved assessment techniques, research protocols, and methods of data collection. Varieties and amounts of data obtained increased dramatically. Large amounts of data also became available as space technology was directed to human health problems. Physicians came to be assisted by specialized engineers, technicians, respiratory therapists, and nurses who provided observations and data that required new models of assessment and analysis.

Mathies cites three structural outcomes of rapidly emerging technologies in medicine. First was the problem-oriented record (POMR) as a systematic approach to medical management. Its components included the data base, the problem list, the initial plan, and the progress report. POMR facilitated the utilization of large amounts of information by the many individuals caring for a patient over time. Second, sub-specialities developed in critical care. As machines become more complex, engineers, computer scientists, and technicians with special competence in the care of machines were required in care settings. Physicians, nurses, and therapists were trained to interface these specialties in the management of critically ill patients. Critical care services required a multidisciplinary team approach to care. Third, life-support technology forced a rethinking of medical curricula. Content on humanism and ethics was included in medical education. Veatch (1977) concurs on factors that resulted from life-support technology. Students were exposed to content on death and dying, human behavior, family-patient relationships, medical ethics, and philosophy in education and practice areas of the medical school curricula.

The literature in critical care nursing in the decade of the 1980s reflected concerns about the particular outcomes of high technology on both nurses and patients in the critical care setting (DeCrosta, 1985; DeVisser, 1981; Rudy, 1986; Sinclair, 1988; Tisdale, 1986). Specialty and general nursing literature have reported frequently on strategies for coping, monitoring, or adopting new technologies such as dialysis, coronary care, computers, and new machines and monitors (Birckhead, 1978; Brown, 1970; Carnevali, 1985; V. Henderson, 1985). As critical care units have become more common, the specific issues of touch, empathy, and stress, and human problems caused by the highly technical critical care environment, have become more apparent in the literature.

The stress effects of critical care settings have been increasingly recognized. Patients, their families, and nurses are influenced by many factors related to the environment and treatment options in critical care. Stress has been recognized as an outcome of highly invasive and technical treatment since the early 1950s. I. L. Janis's study (1958) of the effects of stress on patients confronted with the unknown dangers of surgery found that careful, appropriate preoperative communication that allowed the patient to rehearse the danger situation mentally could greatly enhance postoperative adjustment. R. J. Vanson, B. M. Katz, and K. Krekeler (1980) reported significant stress effects in patients who witnessed invasive, technical procedures on other patients in a coronary care unit (CCU). Auditory and visual stimuli that increase stress effects in patients who witnessed the routine CCU procedure of Swan-Ganz catheter and pacemaker insertion and cardioversion may be reduced by providing glass-partitioned or private rooms (Vanson, Katz, and Krekeler, 1980: 454–497).

V. S. Wilson's study (1987) of stressors related to patients' psychologic responses to the surgical ICU found that over 50 percent of the subjects had an impaired psychologic response while in the ICU. One third of the sample experienced hallucinations, especially visual, without loss of orientation. Too much noise, losing track of time, hearing doctors or nurses talk about rather than to the patient, and being examined by several doctors and nurses were the most significant stressors that impaired healthy coping. Wilson recommends measures to prevent or minimize excessive stressors such as decreasing ICU environmental noise levels by reducing alarms and ventilator noise and providing private rooms; to detect and treat abnormal psychological responses through regular mental status examination of patients by nurses; and to assist the patient with excessive stress to re-adapt and maintain stability by explanations and continuous orientation by nurses (Wilson, 1987: 267–273).

Wilson and others have demonstrated strong correlations between sleep deprivation and impaired stress responses to the ICU environment. Sleep deprivation is difficult to test as an isolated variable because many factors impair stress responses, including the patient's age, severity of illness, psychological history, metabolic and drug factors, and the use of the cardiopulmonary bypass pump, as well as those environmental factors identified earlier by Wilson. Nonetheless, it is usually grouped with potential stressors and is considered a major factor in patient disorientation in ICU by most researchers (Helton, Gordon, and Nunnery, 1980: 464–468).

Families, particularly spouses or significant others of patients in ICUs, experience a great deal of stress related to the crisis of hospitalization. As B. L. Fife (1985: 108) notes, the serious illness or hospitalization of a family member presents a threatening crisis for a family unit. High levels of stress increase the family's vulnerability to the development of secondary problems related to economics, child behavior, child care, or disrupted role expectations. While some families have the resources to remain integrated during such a crisis, others experience temporary periods of disorganization, and still others are unable to remain intact.

The fear of losing a loved one through death and the stress of the strange and threatening environment of the CCU may precipitate a state of disequilibrium and crisis in family members. Stresses experienced by spouses of heart attack (acute myocardial infarction, AMI) patients in a coronary care unit were studied by M. S. Caplin and D. L. Sexton (1988: 31–40). The spouses and nurses ranked potential CCU stressors. While the two groups gave comparable responses with regard to highly ranked stressors, nurses over- or underestimated several stressors of importance to spouses. Spouses and nurses agreed on the high stress potential of fear of death, seeing the spouse sick, dealing with the ill spouse's reaction to the idea of having a heart attack, and not being informed about changes in the patient's condition. Nurses underestimated the importance to the spouse of trying not to upset the ill person, thinking about difficulties when the patient gets home, not being able to sleep, being lonely, having difficulty concentrating, and the fact that parking was inconvenient and expensive. They overestimated the importance to spouses of indecision by doctors and nurses about diagnosis and lack of satisfaction with answers to questions by doctors and nurses. They also overestimated the importance to spouses of noisy alarms on the heart monitor, the care the patient was receiving, being asked to leave the room for a time, and hearing of another patient's death.

The major implication of this study is for nurses to recognize and to address the stresses experienced by CCU patients and their spouses. Caplin and Sexton make the following recommendations. The nurse can help relieve some of the stresses of fear of spousal death by providing support and encouraging expression of feelings and fears. Continuity of care can help establish a relationship conducive to this kind of communication. Other family and clergy may assist in this process. The nurse should set aside time each day, away from the patient, to communicate with the spouse and to answer questions. Honest information presented in a simple and clear manner will help decrease anxiety. Visiting policies, especially, should be explained clearly at the time of admission. Spouses may be helped to sleep at night by being encouraged to call the CCU at bedtime to check on the partner. Finally, nurses can help by explaining clearly the normal adjustment to having a heart attack. Spouses may worry less if they recognize that the patient's disturbing behavior likely will be temporary.

Stress and coping in families of the critically ill are described by S. L. King and F. M. Gregor (1985: 48–51) in their review of the literature. Although they acknowledge variability due to individual response, their evidence seems to indicate that stress increases when the person has no anticipatory preparation time, when exposure to stress is prolonged or multiple stressors occur concurrently, when events are ambiguous or uncertain, and when the exposure is to an event that involves a life event of importance, such as critical illness or survival. Families of critically ill patients experience high levels of stress not only because of the critical illness of the patient but because the illness or injury is usually unexpected, has an uncertain outcome, and has a critical phase that may be prolonged for days or weeks.

Sources of stress for family members are varied, but include fear of death, chronic pain, or permanent disability of the ill family member; uncertainty about the prognosis; loss of a strong family member; conflicts about the usual roles and obligations of work, dependence, and financial concerns; being away from home, staying in unfamiliar lodging, and loneliness; and the environment of unfamiliar caregivers, equipment, procedures, rules, smells, and sounds. If the patient is unconscious or on a ventilator, the family can experience additional sources of stress. The equipment is proof of the seriousness of the illness, and it prevents the patient from responding verbally. If the patient is unconscious, the uncertainty about outcome and fear of death are heightened.

Family members under stress report somatic symptoms, including the sleep disturbances of sleeping fewer hours and waking frequently, feeling depressed and unable to concentrate, restlessness, loss of appetite, and weight loss. These symptoms may reflect anxiety and/or ineffective coping, where coping is defined as "any efforts at stress management regardless of their effectiveness" (Cohen and Lazarus, 1983: 611). Family members may utilize any number of mechanisms for managing stress. Some of the most common techniques are turning to others for support, remaining near the patient, information seeking, intellectualization, rehearsal, or review of the event, minimizing the situation, repetition, and hope (King and Gregor, 1985).

The critical illness of a patient brings about multiple stressors for family members that they may manage in a variety of ways. Nurses may assist family members to utilize effective coping by helping them identify strategies that have been successful for them in the past and to capitalize on personal strengths and the resources available to them. Further, the nurse can reinforce or support their current effective coping efforts (King and Gregor, 1985: 51).

Many of the stresses of critical care nursing are related to the health care setting as a work environment. High levels of stress seem related to burnout in nurses, which is characterized by physical and emotional exhaustion and a loss of compassion and respect for clients. Burnout is a maladaptive reaction to occupational stressors and may also relate to turnover, absenteeism, serious on-the-job mistakes, and patient neglect (Cronin-Stubbs and Rooks, 1985: 31). Burnout has been discussed in the nursing literature since 1978, and situational and social stressors that contribute to nurse burnout have been reported. These include occupational factors, the work setting, life event changes or personal stressors, and lack of social support. Questions remain about the impact of the intensity and frequency of work-related stressors or nurse burnout. In a correlational-descriptive study to identify stressors associated with burnout in critical care nurses and nurses in other specialties, Cronin-Stubbs found that intensity or perceived impact rather than frequency of job stressors contributes to burnout. For example, the death of one patient in critical care may affect nurses more adversely than the daily pressures of caring for acutely ill patients. Also, significant life events in the presence of high job stress contribute to burnout. The study recommends that critical care nurses control the number and impact of stressors experienced at one time and balance negative with positive changes in their personal and occupational lives. As Cronin-Stubbs notes, "Critical care nurses encountered frequent and intense occupational stressors. Alternating periods of intensity with patients or activities that are less emotionally demanding, such as spending time alone, or decreasing the number of long-term, multi-traumatic patient/nurse relationships per case load, may reduce stress" (Cronin-Stubbs and Rooks, 1985: 37).

J. L. Stehle conducted a literature review on critical care nursing stress. Noting that studies from 1969 to 1972 portrayed critical care units as environments fraught with potential stress for nurses, Stehle questioned: "Where did the realization of critical care stress begin? How does it compare with other nursing stress? and, How active have nurses been in identifying, investigating and alleviating stresses specific to critical care?" (1981: 182–186)

Stehle found that nursing in general was described as stressful before critical care nursing was associated with stress. A 1960 study identified tensions of hospital nursing as patient suffering and death, heavy demands, frightening tasks, and disturbing relationships with patients (Menzies, 1960). In 1965, P. A. Holsclaw identified the following areas of high emotional risk in nursing: the inability to restore patients to well-being and feelings of loss for patients with, for example, kidney transplantation, surgical risk, severe disability, rehabilitation problems, psychiatric difficulties, terminal illness, and critical illness. As early as 1965, writers alerted nursing, medicine, and other professions to the dangers inherent in the "intensively concentrated hospital environment" (Gardam, 1969; Kornfield, 1968; Koumans, 1965; Strauss, 1968; Vreeland and Ellis, 1969).

The early studies and articles all viewed stress as a negative factor, but few authors agreed on a definition of the term "stress." These articles attempted to emphasize the presence of stress in critical care and to identify antecedents to actual stress. Koumans (1965) reported that the two most stressful aspects of one ICU were rapid turnover of staff through rotation and intensity of emotion in interpersonal interaction. Strauss (1968) reported the following stress antecedents for ICU nurses: complicated machinery, a narrow patient care focus, great responsibility, conflicts with the administration, and a crisis atmosphere. Nurse satisfactions related to intimacy, morale, and challenge were also reported. Vreeland and Ellis (1969) noted that patients' physical and psychological conditions were deemed the most stressful aspect of ICU work by nurses themselves. Tensions were described as direct stresses involving patient care and indirect stresses involving environmental phenomena. Vreeland and Ellis made a significant observation about the paradoxical nature of the ICU nurse's situation: warmth and sympathy are expected together with objectivity and assertiveness.

Later stress studies provided schemes for categorizing critical care stresses. C. B. Bilodeau (1973) categorized external stressors into five groups: patients, staff, environment, patients' families, and others. Hay and Oken (1972) identified twelve groupings of stressors: "heavy lifting, cardiac research, unpredictable scheduling, heavy responsibilities, patient anxiety, hectic pace, annoyance by patients' families, severity of patients' illness, lack of ample time off, insecurity, patient personalities, and nurse-nurse conflicts." The categories of stresses in a neonatal ICU reported by M. S. Jacobson (1978) included nurse-physician problems, understaffing, heavy work load, sudden death or relapse of an infant, personal insecurity, and the shock of sight and smells.

Most of the studies reviewed by Stehle reflect both the human response of the nurse to the patient crisis and the nurse's reaction to the structural components of the occupational setting or work relationships. Notably, most of these studies were conducted when ICU environments and patient crises were simpler and less technical than they have become since the early 1970s. The increasing use of ventilators for patient support, organ transplants, cardiac surgery, and the availability of advanced trauma care have increased both the complexity and the ethical dilemmas that health care personnel and consumers must confront. The stresses of these latter factors remain unassessed. A 1982 appraisal of stress and ICU nursing by E. H. Friedman (1982: 26–28) supports his earlier observations (1972: 753) that a sense of mastery and self-confidence can serve as an antidote to stress. According to Friedman, a 1980 survey of stress in 1,800 ICU nurses conducted by J. T. Bailey, D. Walker, and N. Madsen indicated almost complete agreement that the following factors in the ICU caused the most stress: conflict with other health care providers, inadequate staffing patterns, lack of support in dealing with death and dying, inadequate work space and other inefficient factors in the physical work environment, and unresponsive nursing leadership. Interpersonal relationships are the greatest source of ICU job stress (Bailey, Walker, and Madsen, 1980). As Friedman notes, most ICU stress studies indicate that interpersonal relationships in patient care are reported by nurses both as sources of stress and as sources of satisfaction. Further, environmental demands that are appraised by one ICU nurse as stressful may be appraised by another nurse as satisfying or challenging. Friedman proposes assertiveness training for ICU nurses to increase "vigor and self-confidence." He notes that "exposure to high stress with adequate support and skill does not increase the risk of mental and physical illness" (Friedman, 1982: 20).

Rudolf Moos (1984: 334–343) has proposed a model for understanding the crisis of physical illness. Background and personal factors, illness-related factors, and physical and social environmental factors influence cognitive appraisal (the perceived meaning of illness), which influences adaptive tasks and coping skills. Moos proposes that the outcome of the crisis is determined by this process. He notes that the stresses faced by health care staff stem both from the nature of the tasks they perform and the way in which hospitals are organized. Especially in ICUs, the excessive workload and understaffing, fast pace and overstimulation, the lack of time for reflection and minimal control over the pace and organization of daily activities, repetitive activities such as taking vital signs every fifteen minutes, the alertness required to handle complex machines and procedures, and the frequent emergencies are significant stresses for nursing staff.

Other demands and stressors for critical care nurses result from patient care. As Moos notes, "the threat and incessant reality of death, the need to continue full nursing care and involvement with patients with little hope for survival or who are in an unconscious limbo where life is maintained only by machines, forces nurses to confront their feelings about death on a daily basis" (Moos, 1984: 339–340). Other sources of stress for ICU nurses stem from the interpersonal aspects of the nurse's role as mediator and coordinator of the many individuals who come into an ICU each day. These persons include distraught families, frightened patients, and physicians who may cope with their own distress by diverting anger to nurses or by abdicating their responsibility and leaving the nurse to communicate medical issues to the patient's family. Moos notes that when doctors use distancing as their main coping strategy they shift responsibility for the patient's emotional health to the nurses.

As Moos describes, nurses may cope with stress in various ways. The phenomenon of burnout has been discussed previously. Moos notes that health professionals can avoid this "caregiver's plight" by effectively coping with the stressors they experience. Individual coping strategies include constructively using denial (ignoring permanent disfigurement and focusing on a patient's assets), achieving satisfaction from the challenge of a difficult job, using humor, accepting one's own feelings (depression or anger) as natural human reactions, and finding peer support. Organizations can enhance stress reduction by providing support groups and stress reduction resources. Further, hospital policies and structures can be altered to reduce stress. Staffing patterns in critical care can be made more flexible to allow for maximal time off, rest, and periods of temporarily rotating out of high-stress aress (Moos, 1984: 342–343).

Increasing numbers of health care workers recognize the positive effects of exercise and relaxation and are incorporating these behaviors into their lifestyle patterns. Effective communication, assertiveness training and limit setting for and by nurses, and self-care activities can also be helpful (Kinney, Packa, and Dunbar, 1993: 111–112). Nurses and physicians have become increasingly aware of the positive effects of touch, verbal comfort, relaxation techniques, and music in patient care. The outcomes for patients and staff have been the focus of recent studies (Bruhn, 1978; Mitchell et al., 1985; Seaman, 1982; Triplett and Arneson, 1979). Positive physiologic and psychologic measures, including lowered blood pressure, anxiety, and pain, have been reported after the use of therapeutic touch.

New technology imposes both benefits and problems on critical care nurses (Sinclair, 1988). Sophisticated computerized systems provide nurses with highly accurate and precise physiologic measurements, giving a timely picture of the patient's status and facilitating rapid intervention if complications develop. Nurses may receive automatic assessments of chest drainage, urine output, and hemodynamic measures every two minutes. Some computer systems can be programmed to administer blood, fluids, or drugs to patients in small increments based on the computer's frequent assessment of measures of volume loss or changes in blood pressure. Some new technologies replace very invasive, high-risk techniques with less costly and problematic ones. Automation can help the nurse accomplish timely interventions, because critical changes in patient status may occur very quickly and require rapid and accurate decision making.

But technology also has hazards. Patient injury as a consequence of treatment, termed iatrogenic injury, has become a possibility as a result of invasive monitoring techniques. Such risks become even more likely in an era of nursing shortage and entry of inexperienced personnel. In a five-year study N. S. Abramson et al. (1980) found that 25 percent of iatrogenic incidents occurred during July and August, a season typically associated with the presence of new interns, residents, nurses, and other health care personnel. V. Sinclair (1988) notes that the constant introduction of new technology into critical care units compounds the problem of undertrained personnel. Sinclair does not consider another complicating factor that contributes to the hazard of new equipment — the lack of uniformity in the equipment of the new technologies. Free market competition by companies and cost containment efforts by hospitals add to the constant change in critical care settings.

The highly technical ICU environment has received the attention of writers concerned with the impact of technology on nursing practice. P. A. DeVisser (1981: 26–29) notes that the coordination inherent in providing twenty-four-hour nursing at the bedside can reduce the various problems of fragmentation of care, including contradicting therapies prescribed by multiple members of the health team. Further, the nurse can assess subtle subjective changes in a patient's level of consciousness, which technology cannot do. Finally, the nurse must take the continuous data both from technology and from human observation, and then assess and act on them appropriately.

As Susan Blackburn (1982: 1708–1712) observes, in her examination of the neonatal ICU as a high-risk environment, concerns related to re-source allocation, appropriate intervention, and treatment decisions are always present in these areas. The application of advanced technology that helps more infants survive is costly in material and human terms. Caretakers must deal with the constant bombardment of stimuli, the demands to perform very highly technical tasks, and the constant moral and ethical issues related to the use of extraordinary technology. Consumers must confront the cost of salvaging smaller and smaller infants in terms of equip-ment, personnel training, and the cost of long-term care of infants who may have physical, mental, and emotional handicaps as a result of surviving treatment. The developmental, financial, and emotional costs to families and to the infants as they grow have yet to be fully discerned, as does the impact of a high-stress environment so early in life on infants who survive.

Technology, especially computers, influences nursing care. Loretta Birckhead (1978: 16–19) has found that computer operation and paper-work require more of the nurse's time than combined patient care areas of teaching and counseling, talking with family, nursing care planning, and socialization with the patient. Only three areas — basic nursing care, special treatments, and consultation — required more nursing time than the com-puter. Birckhead raises the following concerns that she believes nursing must consider as technology increasingly becomes a part of patient care. As expensive equipment is introduced into patient care areas questions of corporate profit versus patient interests may arise. Guidelines for raising questions in these areas are unclear. Nursing, as yet, has not designed safeguards to protect its role with patients as new technology is introduced in patient care and accepted as if "it is an improvement on the old" (Birckhead, 1978: 19).

Doris Carnevali (1985: 10–18) outlines responsibilities of nurses with regard to technology. The nurse must know patient phenomena that re-quire the use of specific equipment, know expected outcomes as patient and machines interact, know how to operate machines safely, and recognize patient cries that indicate effective or ineffective uses of equipment. Car-nevali does not deal with the morality of equipment use. She accepts the "goal" of technology and advises nurses to adapt themselves to the equip-ment.

In her study of the relationship between nurses' empathy and technology, J. Howard Brunt (1985: 69–78) lists stress, burnout, dehumanization, and fragmentation as adverse effects of technology. Brunt believes that nursing care is based on providing a therapeutic interpersonal relationship with empathy as a primary ingredient. Because technological environments are fraught with obstacles to interpersonal openness and communication, the effect of nurses' empathy, especially in ICUs, is an important issue. In Brunt's comparison of empathy responses of nurses from four clinical units as varied as rehabilitation and surgical ICU, the surgical nurses perceived that they worked in a more technical unit than the other nurses, but all nurses scored very low on an empathy scale. Brunt notes that her results deviate from those of other investigators, where nurses were found to score average to high in empathy, but recommends that nurses should be taught content on empathy in nursing schools and in continuing education offerings.

Policy decisions regarding resource allocation for heroic medicine versus prevention continue to be debated in state and federal arenas ("The Dracula of Medical Technology," 1988). Perhaps the most recent widely publicized controversy surrounding advances in medical technology is the artificial heart debate. Since 1982, when Barney Clark received the "Jarvik-7" artificial heart, the artificial heart has been implanted in four other persons. The machines were crude, quality of life for all these patients was very poor, and all the patients have died. In addition, other mechanical devices that boost the heart (left ventricular assist devices) and are used to support patients awaiting heart transplant are not without their own high risk of complications. Taken together, these machines bring limited benefit to very few at very great cost.

The media attention focused on the use of the "Jarvik-7" seems to imply that the use of artificial organs is somehow new. In fact, the first artificial organ, the kidney dialysis machine, is now forty-six years old (Cauwels, 1986). Other artificial devices and drugs that support natural organic or sensory functions include items as varied as dentures, eye glasses, hearing aids, artificial limbs, and insulin, estrogen, testosterone, or thyroid hormone. Artificial organs are significant in the context of this discussion because of the philosophical issues they raise — prevention versus treatment, resource allocation, and public policy decisions about funding for prevention, research, and treatment programs. Questions of scarce resources for a few versus prevention or care for many remain active public health and policy issues.

Problems related to overdependence on technology include a decline in clinical assessment skills; machine error; inability to detect errors, "trouble-shoot," or repair faulty equipment; and the legal implications of contradictory computer data (Sinclair, 1988). Increased liability, increased stress, and depersonalized care have been outcomes of a highly technical environment. As Ellen Rudy and Donna Lee Bertram (1986) point out, in addressing the trends in biomedical technology toward new knowledge, new technology, and increased costs, sophisticated machines have begun to assume many functions formerly controlled by human workers because machines can be programmed to perform more accurately. Technology also presents copious amounts of data, more than can be fully interpreted. The crux of the challenges of efficacy and efficiency is testing new ideas and discarding old methods that no longer apply. In their discussion, however, Rudy and Bertram present technology as a panacea. They do not consider the realities and constraints of rapid change, the economics of cost containment, and the complex demands of the critical care environment. The critical care unit was not developed as a controlled laboratory for scientific testing of new technologies. The realities and values of that setting are not a controlled technological environment.

Sallie Tisdale (1986) addresses the complexities and subtleties of this critical care environment in a poetic reflection:

> They want help, these people. So do I. We need help in answering certain fundamental questions. Help in asking the question in the first place. Our need goes far beyond economic hand-wringing or ethics committees. It demands an acknowledgement of the surreal reality of the sick, and of the maelstrom in which health professionals stagger. The fecundity of the technology, the sheer weight of the machinery cause us to lament, and yet the surf catches us and sweeps us out to sea. We never think to swim back—we've forgotten how to swim. (Tisdale, 1986: 430)

Dolores M. Garlo (1984) also discusses the legal dimensions of contemporary critical care nursing practice. She points out that the scope of critical care nursing practice has generated particular areas of liability. These areas of responsibility often overlap with physician tasks or with former physician tasks. Areas of potential liability include informed consent, patient care activities and the use of technological devices, decisions regarding life-sustaining treatment, and patient protection. The development of critical care nursing paralleled developments in medicine. The evolution of nursing, of which critical care was a part, has broadened the scope of nursing responsibility. This evolution has been judicially recognized, and nurses have assumed increasing liability for malpractice as well as simple negligence.

Garlo identifies three distinct phases in the development of nursing and the evolution of legal regulation (1984: 245–248). Her first phase begins in the 1800s, when nursing was voluntary and no specific training or licensing was required. During this phase, the first nursing schools in the United States, based on the "Nightingale model," opened in 1873 in New York, Connecticut, and Massachusetts (Kalisch and Kalisch, 1986). Nursing schools increased in number during the early 1900s, and hospitals used nursing students, rather than graduates, as a cheap source of labor. In fact, nurses were not employed in hospitals in any numbers until the 1930s and later, at the onset of World War II (Kalisch and Kalisch, 1986; Melosh, 1982). The first professional nursing organizations were organized in the early 1900s, and members lobbied for registration or state control to provide quality standards for patient care. The U.S. Supreme Court had already recognized the power of states to regulate mandatory occupational licensure (Garlo, 1984).

Garlo's second phase of nursing history was precipitated by the passage of the first nurse registration act by North Carolina in 1903. Every state had a registration act by 1923. The first practice act was passed by New York in 1938. The scope of nursing practice was first defined in terms of specific functions that the nurse was allowed to perform. Since physician practice had been previously defined, the focus of defining nursing practice centered on differentiating it from the practice of physicians. Labor issues came to the forefront during this period. The hospital lobby eclipsed both the drive for increased economic benefits for nurses and the rights of nurses to bargain collectively (Garlo, 1984: 246).

By the 1950s, nursing practice had progressed beyond the existing nurse practice acts. Many nurses were already active in the acts of observation, data collection, and decision making regarding methods of patient care. Although the physician continued to prescribe treatment, the nurse determined the most appropriate way to implement care for a particular patient. Although the American Nurses' Association proposed a model definition of nursing to reflect current practice, independent judgment remained legally unrecognized.

The third phase of legal history in nursing occurred in the mid-1960s, with a shift toward medical specialization (Garlo, 1984). The locality rule, first established in 1880 in Massachusetts, was discarded in 1968 by the same court that created it. A national standard of care for a specialty practice was imposed. Under the locality standard, a patient with chest pain in a rural area received the best care that the small hospital or physician could deliver. With the introduction of a national standard, the specialty standards of cardiology were imposed in all circumstances and settings. Health care was becoming a huge industry, and hospitals grew as employers and as businesses as a consequence of the enlarging insurance industry. Furthermore, the increase in medical specialization decreased the numbers of general practitioners and created a gap in primary care. Nursing responded to this crisis by placing practitioners in clinic settings. These nurses were, in fact, often diagnosing and treating patients in direct violation of nurse practice acts.

Medical specialization also had begun to impact hospital care, and nursing specialization in hospitals paralleled the development of medical specialties (Garlo, 1984; Simon, 1980). The development of coronary care units and intensive care units placed hospital nurses in the same violation of practice acts as the nurses in primary care, including making diagnoses and differentiating signs and systems for the purpose of initiating treatment. Many state nursing and medical associations attempted to resolve this dilemma, but laws in some states continued to prohibit nurses from diagnosing or initiating treatment in any circumstances, despite long-standing acceptance of this reality by both medicine and nursing.

As Garlo (1984: 250) notes, nursing throughout its development has consistently expanded its role into the domain traditionally defined as medicine as a result of unionization pressures, improved curricula in schools of nursing, and rapid advances in medical knowledge and technology. Further, nurses in these expanded roles provide services that are more cost effective than are some services provided by physicians. With consensus of approval by medicine and nursing, general duty nurses "elicit and record health histories; interpret selected laboratory findings; make diagnoses in certain situations; choose, initiate, and modify selected therapies in selected situations; provide emergency treatments; and make prospective decisions regarding treatment in collaboration with physicians" (Garlo, 1984: 251). Critical care nurses routinely perform all these tasks formerly initiated only by physicians. Garlo argues that this redefinition in roles warrants legal recognition.

This redefinition process actually took place in Georgia, following a ruling in early 1988 by State Attorney General Bowers that only physicians could diagnose and treat patients. The law had been passed in an effort to keep optometrists from operating with lasers, decreeing that only physicians, veterinarians, dentists, and podiatrists could "perform any surgery, operation, or invasive procedure" using any mechanical means to cut or alter either human or animal tissue. The law in effect made many routine nursing tasks, such as giving an injection, initiating an intravenous line, or wound care, illegal. The law threw the entire health care community into confusion, and was finally ruled unconstitutional by the Georgia Supreme Court in its 1992 session (Headlines Editor, 1993: 9).

The earliest critical care units were postoperative recovery rooms. As described by Florence Nightingale in 1859, "it is not uncommon, in small country hospitals to have a recess or small room leading from the operating theater in which the patients remain until they have recovered, or at least recovered from the immediate effect of the operation" (1859: 89). The concept of grouping very ill patients close to the nurse for observation and care is often attributed to Nightingale (Hilberman, 1975; Kalisch and Kalisch, 1986). The development of critical care units coincided with developments in medical technology and medical specialization. Trauma care during World War II and the Korean and Vietnam wars refined medical and nursing skills. Advances in mechanical ventilation, notably the iron lung, and parallel developments in immunology and microbiology revolutionized treatment and prevention of poliomyelitis (polio). Soon, concepts that had been successful in the treatment of respiratory effects of polio were applied to the treatment of patients with varied pulmonary diseases, such as asthma, acute pulmonary edema, and respiratory failure. A group of life-support techniques became refined and generally available in the 1960s. These techniques included prolonged endotracheal intubation and mechanical ventilation, closed chest cardiac massage and defibrillation, continuous electrocardiographic monitoring, electrical and drug reversal of cardiac arrhythmias and electrical pacemaking, bedside cardiac catheterization with flow-directed catheters, analysis of respiratory gases in arterial and mixed venous blood, intra-aortic balloon counterpulsation, hemodialysis, and hemodynamic monitoring. Recovery rooms were soon followed by respiratory, coronary, neurosurgical, renal dialysis, and cardiac surgical care units (Ayres, 1984; Hilberman, 1975; Simon, 1980).

The nursing shortage in the United States following World War II was another factor that contributed to the development of intensive care units. Prior to the emergence of the intensive care unit, all hospital patients were cared for on the general ward, in rooms with one, two, or more beds. Open wards with ten to twenty beds were common, especially in public and military hospitals or in sections of private hospitals designated for indigent care. The sickest patients would be moved closest to the nurses' station or would be cared for by a private duty nurse. According to Barbara Melosh (1982: 187), hospital administrators saw the early intensive care units (ICUs) as a solution to staffing problems and as a model of efficiency. Fewer nurses could care for more patients, private duty nurses would become obsolete, and highly skilled workers and equipment would be concentrated in one area. Managerial expectations were short-sighted, however. Staffing requirements both in the ICU and in the wards increased as medical intervention and treatment became more complex and sophisticated. The ICU development occurred as much in response to an enlarging capacity for expert care as for economic reasons. As Charles Rosenberg (1987) notes, "one can hardly understand the evolution of the hospital without some understanding of the power of ideas, of the allure of innovation, of the promised amelioration of painful and incapacitating symptoms, through an increasingly effective hospital-based technology."

The intensive care units of the early 1950s were similar in a number of features, although they developed independently in different parts of the country. Many were located in small quarters that had been hastily converted to ICU care. Although both medical and surgical patients were admitted to the units, surgical patients were in the great majority. In fact, many units were planned to care for patients having specialized thoracic or cardiac surgery and neurosurgery. The ICUs were open wards, with beds separated by a screen or curtain, with equipment crowding the cramped floor space. Visiting privileges were limited or absent. Staff learned on the job and traditional nursing skills provided the foundation for care (Simon, 1980: 4).

The ICU concept was adopted by hospitals very quickly and changes in physical design and total environment were incorporated as ICUs became increasingly common. Many units opened at about this time in many places; in fact, a number of hospitals claim the "first" ICU or CCU. Of these, the Rhode Island Hospital, which in 1955 opened the first ICU in a working space that was specifically designed for ICU use, provides an appropriate case for examining the environmental changes that were incorporated in the early ICUs. The Rhode Island Hospital unit was specialized in that it only admitted surgical patients. It was larger than the first units, with twenty-eight beds organized into four working areas. Most of the patients were in private rooms, under direct visual surveillance of the nurse from the central nursing station. The private patient rooms had outside windows and had "piped in" oxygen and suction. Each unit had a blood pressure manometer on the wall. A physician house officer was present in the ICU at all times, and a room was provided as sleep space for this physician. Special charting procedures were developed, and registered nurses assumed more complex responsibilities, some of which had previously been performed only by physicians. Visiting privileges were liberalized and could be flexible at the discretion of the nurse (Beardsley, Bowen, and Capalbo, 1956).

The design features of the Rhode Island ICU continued to influence later ICUs (Simon, 1980: 4). The physical design, especially private rooms with outside windows, was more considerate of the patient's psychological needs. The scope of nursing practice was broadened, moving into territory previously the prerogative of the physician. The unit design accommodated longer patient stays in the ICU. And greater specialization of nursing skills was fostered, rewarded, and ultimately required. There was evidence that the early ICU had the beginnings of a training program to prepare nurses for the special knowledge and skills required to work in such a complex unit, but little detail exists about this preparation.

As the environments of acute and psychiatric hospitals have gained the attention of environmental psychologists, research has emerged in three major areas (Winkel and Holahan, 1986). The first studies that examined the effects of the physical layout of hospital space on social interaction concentrated on balancing patients' needs for social contact and privacy. From these studies have come current cubic and circular hospital designs. Many of the designs that facilitate nursing observation interfere with patient privacy. Recommendations from these types of studies have resulted in such details as private/semiprivate rooms, lounge areas for visitors and nursing staff, patient bathrooms designed with privacy in mind, and play rooms for children and adolescent patients.

Second, studies have focused on the stressors in the environment, especially levels of stimulation for patients and staff. Studies have examined the effects of varied levels of information and sensory input on patients and staff. The impact of stress on patients, families, and nurses in critical care settings has been discussed previously in this chapter. The stress studies also generated data that have been used to alter environmental stimuli. Lighting, noise, and noxious stimuli have been altered in the design of ICUs. Muted lighting, soft music, clocks, color, doors that close, calendars, windows, conditions that enhance sleep, and the presence of personal possessions are just a few examples of this phenomenon. Similarly, attention has been directed to monitoring information overload for patients in high stress areas so that appropriate information may be received and incorporated effectively.

Finally, studies have dealt with the needs and abilities of patients to exact personal control over information access and the details of the hospital experience. Hospital care has shown steady trends toward participatory styles of care and patients' rights. In fact, studies indicate that patients who exert choice and control experience better morale and improved health status (Winkel and Holahan, 1986: 11–33).

The conflicts experienced by patients in attempting to deal with hospital environments are perhaps best expressed by Norman Cousins in describing his recovery from a heart attack (Cousins, 1979). He cites the following stressors: lack of respect for basic sanitation, the high risk of exposure to infectious agents, and the overly extensive use of x-ray and other technical equipment. Admitted to an ICU, Cousins was bemused by the "circular paradox to intensive care units . . . where patients are provided with better electronic aids than ever before for dealing with emergencies that are often intensified because they communicate a sense of imminent disaster" (Cousins, 1979: 133). Concluding that "a hospital is no place for a person who is seriously ill," Cousins left the hospital and entered a hotel room for peace and quiet at about one-third the cost.

Nurses have a profound impact in shaping the hospital environment for patients (Moos, 1984: 189–194; Noble, 1982: xvi; Charles Rosenberg, 1987: 8–9). As Rosenberg notes in his study of the rise of the hospital industry, patients and families have come increasingly to depend on strangers to care for loved ones in illness and death: "Perhaps the most important single element in reshaping the day-to-day texture of hospital life was the professionalization of nursing. In 1800, as today, nurses were the most important single factor determining ward and room environment. Nursing, like professional hospital administration and changed modes of hospital financing has played a key role in shaping the modern hospital" (Rosenberg, 1987: 8–9).

As Mary Anne Noble (1982) notes, the environment of patients has always been the nurse's concern. Nurses "control" the patient's environment by shaping, changing, developing, creating, and maintaining various details. Noble believes that the nurse perceives the fluctuations of daily routines and their effects on patients because of caring for patients around the clock. The nurse may create a therapeutic milieu or may manipulate factors in the environment to a therapeutic outcome. Thus, the environment of patients has become the special concern of nursing.

Rudolf Moos (1987: 189–194) elaborates on specific measures that nurses and other hospital staff can employ to humanize the hospital environment. These efforts include allowing patients to participate in their own care and to control as many details of care as possible, placing patients in private rooms or cubicles for privacy, turning down the lights at night, scheduling procedures so patients can have free time, keeping monitors out of patients' rooms, and providing a more normal and cheerful environment through the use of color on walls, linens, and curtains. Further, a sense of personal identity can be promoted by allowing patients adequate space, privacy, and personal belongings. Moos recommends attention to both physical and social design so that the beneficial impact of hospital settings may be enhanced.

In the early 1960s, almost a third of patients admitted to a hospital after a heart attack (acute myocardial infarction, AMI) died. Death occurred not from the occlusion of the coronary artery but from the complications associated with it, particularly arrhythmias that interrupted normal electrical conduction, causing cardiac arrest and circulatory failure as a consequence of the failing heart. The technological advances of cardiac monitoring, cardiopulmonary resuscitation, defibrillation, cardioversion, and hemodynamic, biochemical, and metabolic monitoring provided mechanisms of immediate treatment for lethal arrhythmias, cardiac arrest, ventricular fibrillation, and primary pump failure. Principles from these technological advances formed the basis of the coronary care unit. In these units the combined action of special observational techniques, skilled nursing, and specialized medical care prevented deaths from complication of AMI by detecting and immediately treating complications. The earliest units were established in 1962 and 1963 in Toronto; Kansas City, Kansas; Philadelphia; and Melbourne and Sydney, Australia. The implementation of the coronary care unit spread rapidly, revolutionizing the care of the hospitalized patient and the practice of nursing in the hospital setting (Ayres, 1984).

Coronary care units reduced mortality from acute myocardial infarction and improved the treatment of cardiac arrhythmias. These units became the prototype of intensive care limited to a medical specialty. Further, as treatment of primary problems improved survival, patients lived to experience failure of another physiologic system, or to experience iatrogenic problems acquired as a consequence of hospitalization or treatment.

Technology triggered the reality of multi-system instability or failure (Ayres, 1984: xviii). For example, successful treatment of a heart attack might be accompanied by a drop in blood pressure, which could cause a stroke or kidney failure. Often, all systems could be supported with technology until the patient died of massive infection or bleeding, or suffered brain death.

The nurse in the coronary care unit rapidly became the major treatment modality. The nurse was skilled, could implement treatment, and was there twenty-four hours a day. The nurse made electrocardiographic observations, diagnosed the specific types of cardiac arrhythmias, and prescribed electrical and drug therapy, frequently in the absence of physician support. This delegation of major diagnostic, decision-making, and treatment activities by physicians to nurses represented something new (Ayres, 1984). This role change, as we have seen, also placed the nurse in violation of most state nurse practice acts (Garlo, 1984: 249).

The trends in technology, role changes for nursing, and management of complex patients seen in the evolution of the recovery room and coronary care unit occurred in the cardiac surgical intensive care units as improved techniques of cardiac catheterization, extra-corporeal circulation (the heart-lung machine), prosthetic valves and grafts, coronary revascularization, and repair of congenital heart defects made open heart surgery on adults and children safe and effective. Later technologies in the 1970s, 1980s, and 1990s such as the artificial heart and the transplant of single and multiple donor organs, have continued the trends identified above.

The nursing literature in the early 1970s provides two cautionary responses to the intensive care unit phenomenon. Esther Lucille Brown (1970: 21–32) reflected on the implications of the development of intensive care and raised two questions. The first concerned the cost of critical care — the presence of a heavily staffed ICU serving a few patients at the expense of "good care" or regular hospital services. The second dealt with the nature and scope of patient care in the ICUs themselves. The trend toward bringing highly competent staff and patients in close proximity to equipment neglected considerations of the physical environment, patient expectations and perceptions of care, the impact of the environment on nurses, nurse-physician relationships, and the role of the nurse in providing total care. Brown had, in 1948, articulated some of the issues that concerned nursing educators and practitioners as nurses began to assume a more highly skilled and technical role in patient care, especially in assuming tasks previously performed by physicians. Concern at that time was expressed about preparation, competence, and retention of those caretaking and comfort skills considered to be the art of nursing (Brown, 1948: 78–83).

The second note of caution was voiced in 1972 by Julia Munch, the editor of a "Symposium on Units for Special Care." Munch offered the concern that special care not be reserved for the seriously ill patient in a coronary or intensive care unit, a burn unit, or a pulmonary unit to the detriment of the patient receiving intermediate, long-term, self, and home care. Munch made a plea that special care be defined as individualized care and that this care be delivered to all patients (Munch, 1972: 311–312).

By mid-century the American Nurses'Association (ANA) had become increasingly involved with legislative and bargaining issues, and perhaps less involved with clinical practice. Indeed, throughout its history, ANA seems to have been at variance with the views and interests of the practicing nurse (Melosh, 1982). Consequently, clinical organizations grew rapidly and assumed many of the functions of the professional organization. The Association of Operating Room Nurses had been established in 1949 (Flanagan, 1976: 624). The American Association of Critical Care Nurses (AACN) was incorporated in 1969 (Voorman, 1979: 871). Its goals reflected the practice and education issues of concern to nurses in diverse critical care settings. The emergence of AACN paralleled the development of other clinical specialty organizations in nursing in areas such as orthopedics, neurosurgery, obstetrics, pediatrics, post-anesthesia care, and rehabilitation. The fragmentation that resulted has been partially resolved by a late 1970s consortium of clinical organizations with the ANA named the Nursing Organization Liaison Forum. This consortium promotes collaboration and communication between the diverse nursing groups.

Critical care nursing grew rapidly from its roots in the postoperative recovery room. The growth of technology and of medical specialization encouraged a parallel growth in the numbers and types of ICUs. The ICU prototype—a small unit with a mix of medical and surgical patients—can now only be found in the small community hospital. Coronary care units (CCUs), medical ICUs (MICUs), and surgical ICUs (SICUs) are standard in most community hospitals. In major teaching and medical centers, specialty ICUs of every type exist, including pediatric, renal, burn, respiratory, neurosurgical, heart surgery, and organ transplant ICUs, in addition to the CCU, MICU, and SICU. The trend toward highly specialized units continues. Furthermore, the newer ICUs reflect changes in focus from acute care to include trauma, rehabilitation, chronic, and long-term care. Patient stays in ICUs may range from several days to many months.

The nurse emerged as the major treatment modality in the evolving critical care unit. Nurses incorporated many roles, some that had been the purview of the physician and some that were new to both medicine and nursing. While many technical support occupations evolved in health care, nursing continued to incorporate the highly complex skills brought about by technology and specialization into the traditional caring role. Nursing assumed the responsibility for training nurses in critical care skills in the hospital rather than in the academic setting, although graduate education in critical care also developed as a way of preparing clinical nurse specialists, and critical care content began to be included in undergraduate curricula in some programs.

As critical care units became common in hospitals, concerns about the impact of high levels of stress on patients, families, and nurses began to emerge. The invasive and highly technical nature of the environment, the dehumanizing aspects of care, and the outcomes of the care itself—that is, recovery, death, or debility—were found to cause high levels of stress. Concerns continue to be raised about the influence of these pressures on attrition of nurses from hospital nursing.

The United States has experienced a relative and actual nursing shortage since World War II. Various efforts to increase numbers of nurses through increased federal nurse training dollars have had a positive effect. However, increasing numbers of nurses are needed in complex critical care, and acute and non-acute ambulatory, chronic care, and home care, settings. Fewer women have entered nursing as a career because of increasing opportunities in other disciplines with greater opportunities for status and salary (Georgia Nurses' Association, 1988). This loss of nurses through attrition, whether from stress, low status or income, or increased opportunities elsewhere, merits study.

Little is known about the details of the experiences of the practicing nurse as critical care units evolved. Interviews with nurses involved in these settings reveal many insights into the roles of nurses, the scope of nursing practice, the stresses of the settings and the care, and the uniqueness of the nature of interactions of nurses and patients. In Margaret Mead's words, the nurse protects "those in danger . . . from illness, from strain, from shock, from sorrow, from grief" (Mead, 1956). Interviews with critical care nurses may provide data about the precise nature of how they learned to do that as critical care settings evolved.

2. "High-Tech" Nursing: The Contemporary Critical Care Unit

The environment of the critical care unit and the role of the nurse in that setting are portrayed by Hay and Oken:

> A stranger entering an ICU is at once bombarded with a massive array of sensory stimuli, some emotionally neutral but many highly charged. Initially, the greatest impact comes from the intricate machinery, with its flashing lights, buzzing and beeping monitors, gurgling suction pumps, and whooshing respirators. Simultaneously, one sees many people rushing around busily performing lifesaving tasks. The atmosphere is not unlike that of the tension-charged strategic war bunker. With time, habituation occurs, but the ever-continuing stimuli decrease the overload threshold and contribute to stress at times of crisis.
>
> As the newness and strangeness of the unit wears off, one increasingly becomes aware of a host of perceptions with specific stressful emotional significance. Desperately ill, sick and injured human beings are hooked up to that machinery. And in addition to mechanical stimuli, one can discern moaning, crying, screaming, and the last gasps of life. Sights of blood, vomitus and excreta, exposed genitalia, mutilated, wasting bodies, and unconscious and helpless people assault the sensibilities. Unceasingly, the ICU nurse must face these affect-laden stimuli with all the distress and conflict that they engender. As part of her [sic] daily routine, the nurse must reassure and comfort the man who is dying of cancer; she must change the dressings of a decomposing, gangrenous limb; she must calm the awakening disturbed "overdose" patient; she must bathe the genitalia of the helpless and comatose; she must wipe away the bloody stool of the gastrointestinal bleeder; she must comfort the anguished young wife who knows her husband is dying. It is hard to imagine any other situation that involves such intimacy with the frightening, repulsive, and forbidden. Stimuli are present to mobilize literally every conflictual area at every psychological developmental level.
>
> But there is more: there is something uncanny about the picture the patients present. Many are neither alive nor dead. Most have "tubes in every orifice." Their sounds and actions (or inaction) are almost nonhuman. Bodily areas and organs ordinarily unseen are openly exposed or deformed by bandages. All of this directly challenges the definition of being human, one's most funda-

mental sense of ego integrity for the nurse as well as patient. Though consciously the nurse quickly learns to accept this surrealism, she is unremittingly exposed to these multiple threats to the stability of her bodily boundaries, her sense of self, and her feelings of humanity and reality.

To all this is added a repetitive contact with death. And, if exposure to death is frequent, that to dying is constant. (Hay and Oken, 1972: 110)

These observations by two psychiatrists were made in the early 1970s and may seem extreme. Efforts have been made to humanize the critical care environment, but in fact, the critical care setting has become much more complex than that observed by Hay and Oken. But this scenario, because of its date, may well be representative of the experiences of some of the critical care nurses interviewed for this study.

The physical structure and unique function of a critical care unit are as variable as the diverse hospitals in the United States. Many variables influence the characteristics of critical care units. The size and location of the hospital and the characteristics of the population served will influence whether the intensive care unit is small or large, in a rural or urban area, and whether the patients are young families or older, retired adults. The purpose of the hospital also influences the characteristics of the ICU. Small community hospitals have different patient populations than do large, tertiary medical centers. Some of the many criteria for admission include patient age and diagnosis, individual physician practices, community standards, formal criteria of hospital committees, bed availability, and nursing staff availability. Patients are admitted to critical care units for a variety of reasons. These include observation and surveillance of their primary medical condition or its complications, care and treatment of an acute illness or injury, postoperative care, either routine or complicated, and delivery of specialized technological monitoring or treatment (Holloway, 1988: 1–50).

The increasing size of the older adult population is another factor that influences the population of patients served in critical care units. Moreover, not only are patients living longer; they are surviving acute illness that would have been fatal in earlier years. Patients suffering from a chronic illness like diabetes now have extended lives as a result of successful management of their clinical health problems. These various population characteristics result in an older population of patients being treated in critical care units, who may have complicated health histories and repeated exacerbations of chronic health problems. Finally, the politics and economics of health care influence the populations seen in critical care units. Hospitals compete vigorously for those hospital services likely to be lucrative. These include, for example, emergency services and high-technology services such as cardiac procedures, organ transplant, and research therapies. Shifts in services provided by hospitals influence the characteristics of populations in critical care units. Hospitals that provide critical care for the indigent or uninsured, and those covered by various local and state welfare or Medicaid programs, are particularly influenced by the shifts in profitable services away from their hospitals. In fact, many of these hospitals have closed, leaving large populations of urban and rural poor unserved (Holloway, 1988: 16–17).

Several trends influence all areas of health care, including critical care nursing (Moorhouse, Geissler, and Doenges, 1987: 103). The escalating cost of health care has generated several outcomes that have had a broad impact on health care delivery. The prospective reimbursement system for hospital Medicare patients, introduced in 1983, and current managed care competition require cost containment measures and a redefinition of minimum standards of care for hospitalized patients. The patient care plan must reflect a strategy that best meets the patient's needs within time restrictions and limited resources. The goal of efficiency imposes shorter hospital stays for patients, restructuring of hospitals for economic survival, and attempts to quantify nursing care costs. Patients in hospitals are sicker, are being treated more expediently, and are being discharged before they are fully recovered from their illnesses. Home health care and ambulatory services are mushrooming in response to the need and the economic incentive (Freeman et al., 1987).

A second trend in health care relates to the highly technical hospital environment (Moorhouse, Geissler, and Doenges, 1987: 1–3). Rapidly changing technology imposes both knowledge requirements and a growing concern about the impersonality of the critical care environment. Nursing has responded to these issues by attempts at collaboration and communication in education and practice, innovative attempts at care planning through computerization, organized training and education plans for staff, and new roles and structures in nursing practice (Simpson and Brown, 1985).

Nursing as a discipline is becoming inextricably bound to technology (DeVisser, 1981: 127). Specialization in medical practice since the 1960s has imposed a national standard of medical and nursing care (Garlo, 1984). Prior to that time, a physician might determine appropriate care for a heart attack patient. This care might be influenced by the region, the personal philosophy of the physician, and the resources of the community and hospital. The general practitioner in a small town might have a different standard than would the teaching hospital in a large city. This is less the case now than ever before. National medical board certification now determines obstetric or cardiac care in both urban and rural areas, and these standards are upheld legally for physicians, nurses, and hospitals.

Hospitals in small towns may have equipment and offer services once only seen in a medical center. Regional trauma and neonatal ICU networks illustrate this phenomenon. Third-party payers, including Medicare, impose a further standard for hospital care. Accreditation standards set by the Joint Commission on Accreditation of Healthcare Organizations also promote similarities rather than differences among hospitals. Critical care units have emerged as a common feature of hospitals in the 1990s. The consequences of technology for nursing practice include demands for education and training, the emergence of specialized clinical roles, creative and often expensive staffing patterns, salary incentive programs, concerns about attrition of expert staff, stress and job tension, and the stresses of ethical dilemmas arising in critical care settings.

Critical care nursing, now an expected part of hospital care in the 1990s, seems rooted in two distinct features. First, the magnitude of patient needs calls for twenty-four-hour nursing surveillance. The nature of this nurse-patient relationship has social, structural, institutional, and economic roots in the evolution of nursing in the United States. Private duty nursing and hospital staff nursing both contain elements of this model of nursing care. Second, the critical care unit has emerged as a geographic entity in hospitals, structuring patients and nurses together in response to medical and surgical specialization and increasing technology.

Critical care nursing may reflect other evolutionary changes in twentieth-century nursing. Nursing education has increasingly moved to collegiate settings, and changes in nursing practice include performance of comprehensive physical and psychosocial patient assessments. The emerging trend toward theoretically grounded practice and research has been steady. The practice of critical care nursing is increasingly complex and sophisticated. Further, the consequences of feminist ideology and labor practices in medicine and nursing practice in hospital settings are but two of the social trends that have influenced the larger society as well as nursing as a discipline. Questions about the distinctiveness of critical care nursing practice seem rooted both in past practice settings and in the unique interpersonal and technological environment of the contemporary critical care unit.

This chapter describes these phenomena using the experiences of nurses themselves. Many of these nurses were involved in planning and/or working in the early ICUs and CCUs (coronary care units). They describe the impact of increasingly complex technology and environments on the practice of critical care nursing, particularly the stresses associated with critical care practice. In many cases these issues overlap. Nurses may describe their experiences as stressful and yet satisfying. Technology may be perceived as a blessing, yet the actual and potential outcomes may be painful and dehumanizing. Some of their experiences parallel findings in the literature; others reveal previously unknown dimensions. Here are their views.

Lee Usher, sixty-one and a nurse since 1947, is currently a director of nursing. She was an assistant director of nursing in the early 1960s at a teaching hospital in Atlanta where she witnessed the transition to specialized units from male and female wards and later took part in the planning that preceded the early ICU and CCU:

I came in 1956. I can remember recognizing that it's very hard to practice nursing having as many physicians come to the unit as came to the thirty-two-bed unit. We just had one nurses' station, which was in the middle, and then you had the whole corridor. The traffic and the interactions that you had to have—See, the doctors were becoming more specialized then, you had neurosurgeons, you had orthopedic people, you had a lot of general surgeons. We didn't have plastic surgery in those days; we didn't have psychiatry here then. But we decided that we needed to segregate the services and that's when 6E became what was cancer, or now oncology. And I remember we put neurosurgery on 3West or 3East. I've forgotten which right now. But the neurosurgeon at that time was very much against putting all his patients together because he said he didn't want all of those families in the same place, with their family members for the most part dying, and putting all those people together, and he didn't want it, but nonetheless, this was nursing's initiative. We prevailed and did get the services separated and eye was on 2West, neurosurgery was 3West, cardiology was 4West, general medicine was 5 and 6West, general surgery was 5East, and 6East was cancer, and LEP2 was OB [obstetrics] and nursery, and that's the way we began to do it. I was telling you that the neurosurgeon was very much against it. It wasn't too long that if he had a patient that was not on 3West he wanted them transferred down immediately. He just couldn't go visit everywhere.

The term "off-service" began with that.

That's right, and one of the outcomes of this is that all at once doctors knew who the head nurse was because they dealt with that person for the most part, and those people had their patients and if anything needed to be done the doctor had to consult with the head nurse. So I think that got us closer working relationships between nurses and physicians. We just couldn't be all things to all people, and we couldn't know orthopedics and GYN [gynecology] and GI [gastrointestinal] and all of that. The traffic flow was just one part of it, but the main reason was that we needed to be able to give better care and we needed more knowledge about what we were doing and we couldn't begin to know everything, so that was the main reason for getting the specialty services within the units to the degree possible.

Usher continues to talk about the early development of the intensive care unit:

Well, I'll tell you what, there was something that came before the intensive care unit—3East and thoracic surgery. In those days we were doing pneumonectomies and lobectomies [removal of a lung or part of a lung], and those were pretty serious technological types of procedures and those patients were extremely ill. I guess a pneumonectomy to me is one of the most difficult patients to care for because of the tracheal shifting and so forth that you can get, but with those patients who were having these surgical procedures and who were sick already, we needed to be able to care for them better than we were doing. In the past, if you had a sick, sick patient whose care was beyond the scope of the nurses on the unit, what you did was you hired a private duty nurse. Well, a private duty nurse wasn't able to keep up with all the knowledge that you needed as fast as the technology was increasing, and this is not only with procedures but with medicine and other things too. So we were having a difficult time really giving the needed care to our thoracic surgery patients. Down the hall we had two rooms that had a connecting bath, and there were doors, of course, on the inside of the corridor to the bathroom, and what we did was put a piece of plywood over the bathtub and make us some cabinets or some shelves in the bathroom, and we put us a station in there with all the drugs and all the supplies and a place for the doctor and nurse to sit to chart and so forth, and that way you didn't have to come out into the corridor, and you could observe patients in two rooms. First we had just one patient in each room, and then it was working so well, we began to put two patients in the room, and I remember saying to the surgeon, "I don't know if the patients are going to like being that close together or not," and I remember him saying, "Well, if I tell the patients that it's the best thing for them to do," he said, "I could tell them that they needed to lie on the floor and they would lie on the floor if they thought it was a better thing to do." But that was really our first intensive care unit at that time. Now if other people were doing it, I don't know if we were aware of it. I think we just saw the need and developed it, and I'm not sure that we had ever heard the word "intensive care" at that time, but it was a way of concentrating the patients that needed the care along with the supplies and equipment and the personnel. So that was our first one in 1960.

We began to see that there were more than just those patients that needed close observation and we needed more beds, so we went to 5A, which was then a classroom, if I remember correctly, and it's not a bad unit even today. What we did was build the private rooms on the outside and have the center, core, for the activities to take place and have visibility by putting the glass in, and you could kind of turn around, and it wasn't too far from the nurses' station to any room or from whatever you need to be doing.

What made you plan the private room?

Well, I really think that insofar as the patients were concerned I remember that we had become extremely aware back then that patients who were sick, sick, sick weren't getting a whole lot of rest because of the constant interruptions that we were doing with them, and then if they had to be aware of everything else that was going on, that it wasn't very good for the patients. I guess we planned the private rooms really and truly because of the care of the patient and the reason that, with intensive care, you didn't know night from day that much and the windows would help, and you had to protect patients from other patients and all the care they were getting 'cause if you weren't doing something for this patient you could be doing something for the patient in the next bed, which would be disruptive to the other patients—the nursing care being the greatest denominator there, and then of course concentration of supplies and equipment.

Vera Strickland, fifty-seven, a nurse since 1954 and also currently a director of nursing, was another assistant director of nursing in this teaching hospital and worked with Usher to plan this preliminary ICU in the late 1950s:

The way we got started with a thoracic unit was: thoracic surgery was coming much more into its own, so we began to place all the patients up there. We had very few doctors that did the procedures, and they wanted a unit, and that was also a piece of how units began to get specialized, because the doctors wanted to place their patients all on one unit. They could make better rounds, and they could be more readily available, and they could do more effective teaching, and again, feeling that the nursing staff would know what they particularly wanted for their patients, so the third floor was designated as the thoracic unit. Then, when we started doing some of the surgery, most of those patients, post-surgically, would have private duty nurses. It got to the point where we didn't have enough private duty nurses that really knew how to care for them or wanted to care for them because it began to get more complex.

Nurses were doing a lot of the parameters we now have machines doing. Nurses had to monitor patients very closely to make sure the patient's indicators stayed within certain parameters, and some of it got to where you didn't have a lot of private duty nurses who felt they wanted to do that or they felt comfortable doing that. We had two semiprivate rooms at the end of that hall, each with two beds. Each had its own toilet, but they had a shared bathtub between the two. So we got our heads together and felt like we were having so much difficulty getting private duty nurses to take care of the patients, we kept pulling the staff off, and many times we would put staff on with the post-surgical patients because we didn't have some private duty nurses that were versed in it. Not that they couldn't learn, but that they just weren't versed in the caring of those patients. So we finally got the idea, why not take those two rooms, take the door down between the two that enters into the tub area, put shelving in there, so you could have some supplies, and put those patients after surgery or those that were critically ill in those two rooms, and that was the beginning of our first ICU. And then we employed private duty nurses who had taken care of these patients who were willing to come on the staff and began to strengthen the staff so that we did our own preparation of the nursing staff to be able to take care of those patients around the clock. We were still using oxygen tents at that time, and this was when you were beginning to get more equipment. I hate to tell you this, but we had wires taped all over the floor. Some of these procedures were fairly new. People came to us from everywhere to have them done. We took adults; we took children. I can remember one little fellow that became the sweetheart of the unit. He arrested four times. And to my knowledge that little fellow is still living today. Very unusual, but it got to the place that the nursing staff became very possessive of their patients. They wouldn't let anybody else handle them. They extended themselves beyond extension to take care of those patients because they began to know what you had to watch for and began to know the indicators, began to know what the doctors would think, and even knew so much about some of the cases that they began to be real teachers to the interns and the residents, if they would listen. I can vividly remember seeing a young staff nurse, a super person, with thoracic surgery in care of children, hovering over a little baby. She knew that we had just gotten that child into the parameters where we were fairly stabilized, and the doctor wanted to come and do something, and she bodily covered that child to keep the doctor from doing anything at that point, because she knew that would be something that would tip the scale. Thankfully enough, when the doctor talked to the attending physician he said, "Yeah, don't, don't do anything right now," so you had nurses who were very committed to that, very committed to a high quality of care, very committed to being knowledgeable. They wanted to learn. They wanted to know and were super with it.

Strickland further reflects on the changes that have come with increased technology:

I guess in some ways the only thing I see sort of changing is the technology that supports what we're trying to do, which means you've got to know a lot more because you have got a lot more data coming to you. You've got more precise data because of technology, and you've got to know what you're dealing with. Because of more precise data we're able to do more. We didn't have monitors; they didn't exist when we opened up those little units. So the nursing staff had to look at some other indicators of the patients: vital signs, and that sense that nurses have when things aren't going right, checking things out, being on top of things. You had to use what tools you had, and yet there's always that same aspect of assessing what's going on with the patient, using whatever data you've got you can pull on. Today we've got more technology. We've got more precise data. We've got more technology to support us. Now the nurses can listen for the alarm. They don't have to worry about that in a sense. Whereas the nurse had to be the watcher of something exceeding an acceptable parameter. They had to monitor it. They were the alarm. Now we've got all those supports there so they can begin to look at some other things. As things got more complex, I've probably seen two things. One, nurses wanting to know how to use it, and I think for a period of time maybe nursing, and medicine too, wanted to rely on that in contrast to really looking at the patient. You know, immediately you want to get this laboratory procedure and that laboratory test and so forth and so on, sometimes almost relying too much on that. I don't want to get that out of perspective, but I felt like really saying: What do we need? What is going on with the patient? Almost stopping long enough to do a good assessment of the patient to determine, "Okay, this is what we think is going on. What diagnostic tests, what laboratory procedures do we need to either support that or lead us to what is going on?" Of course, I haven't been in an acute care setting for a good while now, but I'm sensing a little less of that. I don't know, maybe it's still there, but certainly when you've got all this stuff coming to you that was so wonderful you just love to use it. And a little bit of the other was not into play as much, if you know what I'm talking about.

Trish Maddox, fifty-three, has been a nurse since 1951. She was head nurse in the ten-bed thoracic ICU that in 1963 replaced the four-bed preliminary unit described by Usher and Strickland. The focus of the new unit was to accomplish the nursing care that the private duty nurse had done in a specialized unit:

You have to remember in those days there was not as much technology as there is now. And nursing was not as complex. We never thought of the private duty as having more expertise, but it was simply that they had the time because the patient needs were complex. You didn't have a lot of the equipment, like monitors, and nursing was just not as involved because medicine was not advanced, or nursing either. So when I went through nursing school, we weren't even putting pacemakers in. You know that the most complex things you had were oxygen tanks and chest bottles and catheters. You didn't have patients that had arterial lines and things like that. You weren't doing dialysis or open heart surgery. In other words, medical care was a lot more simple. They had IVs, and they got blood. They could have a lot of dressing changes like burn patients. But some of them were more demanding-type patients, the burn patients. Patients in oxygen tents were challenges, because they did use a lot of oxygen tents then supplied by tanks, and trying to take care of a patient with an oxygen tank was really difficult.

Just getting to them was difficult.

Yes, just getting to the patient was difficult. You still do those things today in nursing as far as skin care and things like that. But nursing was simpler from a standpoint of what could be done for the patient. The nurse really had almost direct patient contact then. You did not have the machine between the nurse and the patient as much, except for instances when we had an oxygen tent. But otherwise you were not dealing with as much equipment. You were doing more of the direct things. Checking the blood pressure, dressing changes, bathing, and giving medication. That kind of thing. You were not doing nursing with the equipment.

And if someone was really sick?

Direct observation and the frequency of the care. The person might be unconscious or bleeding. Another thing is immediately post-op. Most patients had a private duty nurse the first twenty-four hours after surgery, especially what we think of as major abdominal surgery, something like that. When they came back to the unit from the recovery room they would still have a private duty nurse. At least for one night.

She describes the opening of the ICU:

Yes, in the fall of '63 was when it opened.

What do you remember about the equipment and the preparations of the staff?

Well, looking back, I feel like that the people that set the unit up physically probably did a good job in terms of the overall supplies. I don't remember what was available back in those days. I think that was probably okay. We had an emergency cart. All kinds of needles and syringes. Just basic stuff pretty much. Dressing trays and things like that. But that was okay. I don't remember anything negative about that. We had ten individual patient rooms. This was the philosophy. The nurse would be in the patient's room and everything would be done from that point. Rather than the nurse being in the middle of the unit she would be in the patient's room.

How did that concept of having the nurse and all the data in the patient's room evolve? It seems unique.

Well, it's probably not as radical in a way if you think about it because when the private duty nurse was taking care of the critically ill patients I remember most of the time they would take the chart to the room and they would put the care plan inside the chart. They were going to be in the room all the time. So they would take the care plan out and put it inside the chart and they would go back to the patient's room and they kept it there all the time.

In a sense that probably was a carry-over from that. I really don't know what factors were coming to bear and what created the need for intensive care units: the need for a group of nurses to be educated to have more specialized knowledge; probably bringing more nurses together. It was a lot of things that came to bear in terms of monitoring and more patients that were ill. Although when I look back on it, there was probably always a need for something like intensive care. I can remember as a student working on the cardiology unit where you had a lot of patients who came in with heart attacks. We would make rounds at night in those rooms just hoping that they would be alive. I can remember we had to go around with flashlights and go into their room. We would go up to the bedside and count their pulse and check their breathing. That was your way of monitoring them. So there was a need then. I'm not real sure why it took so long to bring that concept in. I guess maybe we just didn't have the monitoring equipment—I suppose monitoring equipment was one of the breakthroughs that brought about ICUs. But it's interesting to note that when we opened our ICU we did not open it with monitoring equipment. So I know it was not necessarily the thing that precipitated it at our hospital. Because we did not have any monitors in the units when we opened. All we had was an EKG machine for the unit. It was really still the idea of more direct observations by the nurse. The nurse was closer to the patient. That particular unit was not opened specifically for that purpose because we didn't have any monitors.

The reflections of nurses about the ICU experience in this teaching hospital support the literature. The units were small, increasingly specialized, and created from space not originally intended for that purpose. Betsy Tanner, sixty-one, a nurse since 1947, describes a similar experience in a private community hospital when the first coronary care unit was opened. She describes previous care of very ill patients:

Well, when I was first a nursing student I moved patients many times in the middle of the night in the ward. We kept our more acutely ill patients closest to the station. We had a private room that we came to call our sick unit. It was a two-bed room and you literally, by the way, would have to crawl over the bed almost with some of the oxygen tanks. And all of the large Wangensteen suctions—the big five- or ten-gallon cylinder tanks. You crawl over the equipment or mostly over the patient's bed and the equipment. But we would move patients—you'd lose a patient so you'd bring your next most critical out. So it was a concentration of the observation factor before you had the technology. Then as the technology became available you started adding that. I can remember being summoned to the conference room of our medical director. We were given a copy, as I recall, of the *New England Journal* that talked about how we could decrease the mortality if we established a coronary care unit, and we talked. I don't even recall who else was there, but I'm sure there were others. And we talked about it, and we began to talk about how we could establish such a program. What would it cost and what could we do about the nursing. And I was very interested in the article. And we took our steam room—with the advent of—antibiotics. I'll take you back to my second staff nurse position—in the communicable disease.—In the summer we had polios, the fall and the winter months we had whooping cough, croup, the common childhood diseases, measles, and we got all of the community's childhood diseases. So we got pretty much of the state's complicated childhood diseases. So we had diphtheria and we had a tuberculosis acute care facility. They went up to Rome for convalescence, but when they were running their temps and had meningitis and what have you, the complications so to speak, we brought them to the city hospital and in my first nursing days, I was nursing when we began to get penicillin. Used to give penicillin every hour and then we got the more refined and we lived for the day when we could give it every three hours and then every six hours and then every twelve hours and then daily.

Before antibiotics, we had the steam room. We had a steam room at this private hospital, which was a room adjacent to pediatrics that was tall from floor to ceiling. And we had a steam line and the patients were placed in. At City Hospital, we made croup tents. And we made croup tents out of oil cloth and wool blankets, and the child was concealed. You can see the apprehension and anxiety on behalf of the child to be there as opposed to just be in the steam room. And this was the private hospital that had the steam room, so that sort of puts it into perspective. But anyway, we didn't get croups—we no longer needed the croup room, so we used that room and the other ward part of our pediatric unit here and we just combined that and made ourselves a coronary care unit. I think that was in '66. Maybe. 1965 or '66. I don't recall who else in the city had one—but the irony was the city hospital always had the latest technology first as part of the teaching program.

Finally, Carla Olson, forty-four, a nurse since 1965, now a clinical nurse specialist in cardiology, describes the evolution of the coronary care unit in the same hospital where Usher, Strickland, and Maddox helped found the early ICU:

What was appealing about cardiology in 1966?

The patients were experiencing no rehab, and it was obvious that physically they seemed to have more capacity than the culture or the medical staff or the patients would openly acknowledge, and if there was some way to return them to a more functional status without quite the same fear, then we wouldn't have cardiac cripples. So that was my initial attraction and knowing the technology was there, that we were going to have something different in the way of monitoring them and intensive care in the beginning phases that I know would probably make some difference in the long run, too. It was a very active, crisis-oriented, well I say active. There were plenty of times when it was low level when they were recuperating, but every once in a while you had a real challenge, and I liked that. The patients we had at the time were already having acute events. And the new MIs [myocardial infarctions] were inevitably admitted to the empty semiprivate rooms in the middle of the night. The first day we opened our CCU, the patient who had been admitted in the middle of the night coded [suffered cardiopulmonary arrest] within thirty minutes after I came on duty working on the floor, and he was the first patient that we resuscitated, so it was real obvious that we needed a special place for these people that we could detect the arrest and treat it.

So there were not monitors either?

Well, no, not when I first went over there. We didn't have an EKG machine, and we certainly didn't know how to work one. But it's interesting when we opened the CCU at seven o'clock in the morning that we wouldn't have known that the patient that was admitted at two o'clock in the morning needed to be in there. I mean we just opened officially and were waiting on admissions.

Some formal admissions.

Yeah, right, and this patient that had been admitted in the middle of the night, it didn't occur to anyone to move him over until he coded, and so the first patient that I defibrillated, which was him, the piece of equipment made this extremely explosive noise like a gunshot or a backfiring of a car when I hit the buttons. That particular machine would build up dust, and every six to eight months when you used it, it would just fire away and you had this enormous noise. And the salesperson happened to be on the unit looking over the equipment making sure everything was okay when we had this code and of course he heard the noise. You could have heard it anywhere on the fourth floor. And I thought I would never shock anybody again because I just knew I had done something wrong, and he couldn't figure it out. He had no idea why that noise would have occurred. So we tested the device several times in succession and it never did that again, never. And he had to go back to the factory to come up with some reason that it was doing that. I mean it was at least six months before it did it again to some poor unsuspecting soul. I thought, well, you can imagine never having defibrillated ever, never having any idea what it would do. We didn't even have defibrillators in codes that I remember. I don't remember ever seeing a physician using a defibrillator or anything like that when we had codes, so it was all new to us. The first time I hit the button it was just about the last straw because I thought, well surely I had shocked myself or somebody else or hurt the patient or something horrible had happened because it was just awful. The only medicines I remember were IV narcotics and nitroglycerin of some sort. We probably had Isordil, [a coronary vasodilator] but we didn't have beta blockers or anything like that. A lot of sublingual nitroglycerin. We may have had the ointment but it wasn't used as much as it is now.

The few lectures we had to prepare for the opening of the CCU were done by the doctors. I remember one of the cardiac fellows doing the lecture on defibrillation, and I had every reason to believe that he had never defibrillated a patient in his life. However, he did know the machine, and he was able to tell us what to do with it. But it became obvious that none of them knew anything about what this was going to be, so that they were guessing what we might see once we opened. Really, they had no idea either, so it was like in the dark. Apparently Macon had a CCU for a year or so, and I remember the nursing administrators going there to look at it and coming back with some idea of things, but I don't remember a great deal more about it. But I know the administrators responsible sat down with the cardiologist and got him to chat with them about a few things. I have no idea how they chose equipment or any of that, but it was basically, "Here it is, you develop it." You know, "Here's the structure, here's the narcotics, and here's your fluids, and we'll help you any way we can."

Did your title change then to clinical nurse specialist?

No, I had no interest in changing my title at that point, because we didn't know what we were doing, and it was just learning as you go, and it was extremely stressful for the four of us because we were constantly under the apprehension that something else was going to happen that we didn't know what to expect. The second patient that coded, I think in the whole place, was again on my shift and it was a myocardial rupture. We had no idea what to do for a normal sinus rhythm in a patient with no pulse or breathing. Nobody had even mentioned that as a possibility. We had a programmed response for V fib [ventricular fibrillation] and a programmed response for asystole [cardiac standstill], and that's all that we had any kind of idea about.

So it was a real stressful experience, because you had no idea what was coming next, what the patients were going to do that you didn't know what to do for. So there was a lot of camaraderie between the physicians and the nurses. They were in it with us, but they had no idea. So we learned. Every day was another potential experience or nightmare. The first patient with VTAC [ventricular tachycardia]: we assumed VTAC would be a nightmare, emergency-crisis-oriented kind of thing. And the patient walked up four flights of stairs instead of waiting for an elevator because he had to hurry to get into the hospital. We had the paddles greased. We were expecting an admission on a stretcher that was coding, that type of thing. And the patient walks in with a suitcase. And it was either one extreme or the other, constantly, all the time.

The arrhythmias didn't fit the textbook pictures at all. The variation you had from one patient to the next was totally unaddressed. We thought sinus rhythm was going to look like the textbook drawing. We didn't find anybody that had sinus rhythm that looked like that. So once we realized after the first few days that it was going to be that type of newness every single day, we all had major stress symptoms. I would wake up at night with nightmares and hearing bells and hearing alarms and stuff, and the others had GI distress and headaches, and it was pretty traumatic. Two of the others didn't last but about six weeks or two months.

So we approached the physicians, to train some more people, and they helped us a little bit with the second course. But it was worse than the first because the physicians were just obviously not going to put what time and effort it took into doing it. So I think along about January I said to the assistant director that it was obvious that we were going to have to take over our own training, and by January or February I kind of knew what the problems were going to be, and then I asked to be converted to a clinical specialist and I'm sure that I got that title at that point. The way I implemented it was one-on-one role-modeling in the CCU for training when we had new people, so I was in there all the time. I never left when I had a new person. Then, when I didn't have a new person, I could work more on the recovery phase with the nurses out there on the floor and start patient education programs. That phase of one-on-one teaching lasted until we got the course, which I'm guessing was 1976 maybe. I don't think we got a central training course until we opened up those other ICUs, and we moved in 1975.

So what equipment did you open with in the CCU?

The one defibrillator that made that sound, which I'll never forget, and we had a bedside monitor for each room, and a central station, an alarm to get help from the floor, and a couple of shelves of our own supplies.

Any kind of crash cart?

Oh yeah, uh huh. Very simple though. It's interesting to think back on the physical simplicity of the supplies and the space the supplies took up. Then versus now. It's just unreal. You don't think of it until you really get a picture in your mind of what you worked with, and it was plenty of supplies. You really didn't have a lot of problems running out of things, but we use so much more now of a variety.

What about pacemakers?

I remember external pacing because the bedside monitor had that feature, and I remember that we did it once, and then the patient really didn't have to have it, so it was turned off. We were supposed to know how to do it, but it was never used. It was an impossible thing to keep the nurses trained in because they didn't ever need it, but we did have that external pacing capability. We had one machine that was portable, too, that provided that type of thing, but it died very shortly after I got there, and they never used it again. Transvenous pacing happened since that time, but I don't remember when. I don't remember it even being a particular miracle, but it must have been at the time.

I remember more caution with visitors because prior to all the invasive things that you could do, you treated them with a great deal more kid gloves approach. So I remember some conflicts about families wanting to stay and not being able to stay and wanting to be in the room for long periods when you wanted them to go out and let the patient rest, so there was some control over visiting that was pretty secure. But I know that it was not as rigid as the other ICUs.

We did have some sort of knock-down drag-outs with families who intended to stay and feed and talk and be a part of that patient's experiences, and we resisted that with the idea that it was unnecessary. I have a feeling that it was because we had no beta blockers, nothing to protect the patient from emotional surges, so indeed some kind of constraints on stimuli were absolutely critical if you were going to avoid having any more chest pain. At that point we had no idea by the cardiac cath what they were vulnerable to next. So everybody lived with the possibility of extending their AMI [acute myocardial infarction], and we had Sunday night infarcts routinely after people visited during the day, so my sense is the patient population might have been more local where that could have been a greater factor. At the present time they are 500 miles away from church visitors, so they don't come quite in the same droves. Plus now we have a lot of protection to keep the patient from having increased oxygen demands every time something happens. But we thought we were doing the right thing. It was right at the beginning of implementing some of the bedside sitting and all that MI patients were allowed to do. It became a real interesting challenge for us to see how much we could get away with, if we could let them sit up and do things for themselves in the chair without causing pain. I remember a couple of very elderly physicians who were shocked to death that we had people in pulmonary edema setting up in a chair. They just could not believe it. But they weren't so stupid as to control us and try to make them go back to bed. They were just in awe of what was going on. They were really only consultants. They had no authority over the patients when they were in the CCU. Only the cardiologists had authority there.

And there was nowhere you could go to find somebody to come in and teach you anything like arrhythmia recognition or whatever. That was just not available.

What continued to be appealing about CCU?

Well, that you didn't have to die from a heart attack, that there was going to be some difference in mortality and obviously you'd salvage more people if you could do something about it, so it just fit in very nicely with what I was interested in. Not only was I interested in, once they'd been through the acute experience, in getting them home safely and back to a normal routine, but I was more interested in anything else we could do in the acute phase to get them through it quicker and better.

The technical skills in the CCU part of it were a surprise to me, but no, none of us had any idea. If any of the physicians had any idea, they didn't let on. Intervening with the defibrillator was sort of unbelievable: that anybody would be doing that, much less the nurse. It's kind of like when you read in the paper about the leeches. It's that dramatic. You don't even consider it. You think of that as maybe one thing, and then it branches out into this and that and the other. So it just evolves on you very slowly before you quite appreciate that it's a different role.

Carla Olson's experiences reveal a great deal about how nurses responded to the demands of rapid change, specialization, and increased technology.

The trends in the evolution of critical care nursing seem aptly summarized in a statement by Lee Usher, who was involved in the early planning of the ICU and CCU at the Atlanta teaching hospital:

What are the biggest changes and transitions you've seen in nursing since your first experience?

Well—I guess that—and this is not original with me, others have said it too—but I guess the introduction of antibiotics helped to change how nurses functioned and practiced as much as any one thing. Ah—before the days of antibiotics—and I am not before the days of antibiotics—but I just told you about the penicillin, and then all the "mycins" that came along and whatever. But if you had someone with pneumonia or somebody with an infectious disease, they stayed for weeks and weeks and they had night sweats and they had high, high fevers and you had to sponge them and use alcohol and ice packs and all of those kinds of skills and procedures to nurse the patient through. And we don't have to do that as much as we once did, but you had to—also, the nourishment of the patients because the fevers or whatever, or the infection was so devastating until the patients would lose weight or lose their strength in such a hurry until you had to work real hard to hydrate the patient.

And then all the processing—you see we didn't have—I'm not all that old, but I think it shows you now rapidly we have developed. Just looking at the suctioning—When I was a nursing student at Charity Hospital in New Orleans, we had to make our own Wangensteen suctions, and we did it with tape and with tubes that went into stoppers that went into bottles, and one was longer than the other and one was shorter than the other, and in order to form a vacuum you had to tape the stopper in and whatever. But we didn't have equipment then. It was after the war was over, and this is the unfortunate, or the fortunate, thing about wars is that it brings all kinds of new learning, new experiences, and new technology. I remember being here when the first artificial kidney machine was introduced. There were so many people, so many doctors in that room until you had to stand on tiptoes to even look into the room to see what the machine was like. Now that's one of the fastest changes insofar as technology goes, because when the artificial kidney machine first came into existence, only the physicians could do it. Then pretty soon the nurse was doing it, and then in no time flat the technician was doing it, and now the patient does it. And that's been rapid, that's been something to watch.

Several themes were consistent as nurses spoke about the evolution of the early intensive care units. Increasing specialization, knowledge, and technology precipitated a need for bringing together nurses who had specialized knowledge with patients. The private duty nurse-patient relationship seemed to be the model for this ICU planning, rather than the existence of equipment or technology. Many of the earlier ICUs opened even without cardiac monitors, now considered one of the most fundamental elements of ICU care. The nurse was the monitor in the early units, using traditional hands-on nursing skills, such as taking the pulse and temperature and providing constant surveillance and observation of patient condition and status. Both medicine and nursing were less complex then and often involved more touch and personal, hands-on ministrations and care, such as alcohol baths for persistent high fevers.

As technology and specialized equipment emerged rapidly, the pace of change accelerated. This rapid change had several outcomes. Nurses were eager to learn new skills, but did not forfeit older methods. Nursing incorporated technical expertise into the traditional constant caretaking considered essential to nursing practice. Both medicine and nursing often experienced an over-reliance on technology that at times resulted in a diminished capacity for manual assessment.

Certainly, technology resulted in more data being available for both medicine and nursing. The nurse quickly became the expert in critical care. Since change was constant, there were few experts to teach and establish acceptable standards of practice. Nurses assumed new roles as clinical educators of nurses, patients, and often physicians, and as clinical experts who used clinical judgment to determine appropriate patient care. Nurses often set limits on patients, visitors, other nurses, and physicians in order to protect patients in the critical care unit. In reality, nurses always exercised judgment in hospitals to protect patients from harm or to provide better care. As the nurses in this study attest, in the days before the ICU the sickest patients were moved closest to the nurses' station so that the nurses could give them more continual nursing care. The physical space for the early ICUs was almost always adapted from areas not designed specifically for ICU care, often from space no longer needed because of technological advances. For example, steam rooms used for babies with croup or patients with pneumonia, which were made obsolete by the advent of antibiotics and the availability of humidified oxygen, were often converted to ICUs.

The changes in technology and the new nursing roles were always a surprise to nurses. Defibrillation of the heart, for example, was described as almost unbelievable. Implementation of new technology was similarly unclear and uncharted. The new coronary care unit described by Carla Olson opened waiting for formal admissions. The first patient had been admitted to a semiprivate room at 2:00 A.M. in the usual manner, and was admitted to the CCU only after he had a crisis. Nurses and physicians had good collaborative, working relationships in these specialized units. Both learned together that the technology and the care would increase patient survival.

The skill acquisition in adapting to new technology was additive. Nurses incorporated the new skills into traditional roles. Nurses in critical care have complex knowledge and skills, and they intervene based on that expertise. For example, nurses give drugs or defibrillate the heart based on their assessment of cardiac arrhythmias. Nurses also diagnose cardiac is-chemia (low tissue oxygen level) from an electrocardiogram and notify the physicians, so that immediate intervention can prevent a heart attack or death. The combination of caring, skill, and continual presence was en-hanced by a new aggressiveness in nursing practice in the critical care nurse. This aggressiveness in assessing and intervening with patients based on specialized knowledge was a new concept. It surprised and confounded many nurses and physicians.

The following interview excerpts present many dimensions of the interrelationship between the increasing complexity of the critical care setting and the environment, the nature of the work, and the nurse-patient interaction itself. Lisa Fields, thirty-one, with critical care experience since 1977 in two urban hospitals, describes the impact of technology on her own person and on her interaction with patients and families:

What is satisfying about ICU practice to you?
The level of skill confidence is very satisfying.
What are the frustrations about ICU practice?
It depends on the setting. At this teaching hospital, I think that the staff-patient ratio is much better than at other hospitals. At the community hospital, one night, I remember, I had four very sick ICU patients. You can't take care of that many ICU patients safely at the same time. The reason that I floated in the units was because I liked the level of competency that I could achieve in the unit and, at the same time, I really like the balance. If I were out on the floor I could relate to patients much more on an emotional level. There was just more opportunity to talk to them as people and get involved with them. Whereas in the unit [CCU] it seemed like most of my experiences were with people who were sedated and it is much harder to establish a rapport, although I really enjoy CCU because those people who are back there are the ones that are sick. But they may not be symptomatic, but they are alert and you can communi-cate. I also think another thing that I really enjoy is with the technical aspects of ICU nursing. Sometimes, it tends to separate me; I guess I just let it happen. I have never really thought about it, but it somehow separates me from my identification with the patient. It is harder to identify this patient as a real person when they are always horizontal and I am always vertical. When they have so many tubes and wires and they are restrained or tied to the bed. All of the blinking lights and monitors beeping. All the sounds and lights and other sorts of extra fixtures that are all around them. I guess I just somehow block myself from reality. I find that it must be threatening to me on some level. It is like I am

not as available to them. It also seems like for the most part that they are so scared that I am really dealing with an emotional issue just to placate them or displace their fear. There is really not much more emotional involvement that you have with them other than trying to keep the fear level or anxiety level down. I haven't really found that very rewarding.

I have to say that one of the things that I have found rewarding is being involved with patients' families in ICU because they are in such crisis situations. Especially if you are used to this kind of thing, they just appreciate any kind of support or any extension. I had a patient one time that was at work—he was an elevator repairman and he was in his early thirties. He got his head caught when a hydraulic door closed on him. When we got him he was really in a lot of pain and he was lucky, it was amazing that he survived.

Was his skull crushed?

He had a skull fracture, but he had like this extravasation where his eyes were just pooched out with all this sclera and bleeding from the nose and the ears. He actually lived through it. He was practically a vegetable, but he survived. I remember following him because he would come in for further treatment. He was actually sitting up in a wheelchair. He could almost hold his head up and he was aware of his surroundings, but he could not talk. His wife stuck by him and took care of him. But I just remember every time I would see them I had this feeling of connection with her. I just remember that with several ICU patients who were in crisis where I felt like emotionally I could not do much for them, but they just had to get through it and I will help you in any way that I can. But somehow for me there was more of a profound connection with the family members. I guess that there is an aspect of my personality that thrives on intensity. That is one thing that I get out of the ICU experience. I was totally amazed with my technical skills, that I could work all of these gadgets, and all this business. It became a standard of care almost. Sometimes I would get this thing and think that this was really amazing and at the same time it would be like, wow, look at what I am doing, and then I would have to deal with family members that were hysterical. That was like another crisis situation for me, another situation that I would have to be really up on and interpret that human part of it.

Why do nurses leave nursing?

Frustration. Frustration with exactly what I was describing. I mean I coped with it all the time. I personally could not integrate that level of stress into my life and still feel okay about myself and not be compensated in other areas of my life. I could not do it personally. I don't know how they do it. I would say frustration with the workload, being overworked, being underpaid, being undercompensated, being underappreciated, working holidays—well yes, you get holiday pay, but if you work the holiday, it is not the same when you get July fifteenth off and get paid for the Fourth of July. It is not like even being off. You should be paid extra for working holidays. The hours are stressful, the shift hours. Starting so early, getting off so late. The responsibility of staffing. I have two friends who worked in ICU. One of them was just running her legs off with wedding plans and the other was pregnant. Both of them wanted to work part time, and they wanted to stay with the ICU. They decided that they would approach the head nurse about job-sharing, and she said, no, that there was no precedent for that. They both quit. That is just ridiculous. Personally, I don't like punching a clock. I don't like shift work. I don't like the idea that no matter how hard I work, I am not going to get paid any more. No matter how efficient I am, it is not going to make a damn bit of difference because I am going to have to be there for that period of time, because it doesn't matter. I can do a good job, I can do a bad job, and I will get paid the same and get my two percent raise each year. I won't be able to keep up financially. I won't even be able to buy the same things that I bought last year. It is ridiculous. There is no incentive. There is very little positive influence. Lack of incentive is the real problem. When you get really skilled nurses, with a lot of experience and education, they are accomplished. These are the people that like a challenge. When they have reached their highest level of challenge in a setting, there is no incentive to stay. That is most of the nurses in ICU that I have known. That is me.

What are the support systems in nursing?

Sometimes there is closeness among the staff, but that is potluck. Some staffs work together and support one another. Some do not support each other at all. Support from head nurses is rare. Mostly they become an adversary in this situation. I personally feel that I am extremely unsupported at work, and that is one of the reasons that I choose to work only two days a week. I don't feel support for either who I am as the person or who I am as a nurse. The feedback that I have, the support that I really have as a nurse, is from my patients. I had this little man this weekend who was having an anxiety attack at seven A.M. I stayed in the room and talked to him for about twenty minutes, and I told him I had to leave because the next shift was coming on, and he said, "I will see you tonight, won't I?" I said, "No, I just work weekends." He said he was sorry that he would not get to know me because I was a nice person. It really makes it worthwhile for my patients to give me that kind of feedback. He made a difference. Or for family members to say, "I could not have done it without you." Occasionally, in my experiences, there have been other nurses that have been very supportive, but they are few and far between.

Karen Adler, whom we met in the Introduction, similarly describes her initial impression of the ICU environment and her perceptions of job stresses:

Did you have any experience in ICU as a student?

Yes, as a matter of fact, one of my first clinical rotations was in ICU. Since we were a small group, we spent time one on one with the professor in an ICU setting.

What do you remember about that? That was during the mid-seventies?

Right. I think that one of the main things that I remember was that there was no privacy for patients at all. All six patients were in an open ward setting, and it was just incredible. The stimulation level in there was just overwhelming because there were so many other things happening around you all the time. There would be a code going on three feet away from you while you are trying to take care of a patient. The patient that I was taking care of was a sixteen-year-old fresh quadriplegic, and it was a little overwhelming at first. We did every-thing from— I wasn't at the stage at that point to do injections and that sort of things, but we did all the basic care, bathing, turning on the Stryker frame, range of motion, basic good nursing care that beginning nurses do.

What do you remember as a student about the care of the patient in the ICU?

I remember it being very intense. I remember it to be a real good place where you brought together a lot of the facts that you had gotten from different places. It seemed to all come together real easily in that setting. Other than that, I can't really tell you that it was that much different from the care that I was giving out on the floor other than it was more intense and there was more to be done because you are taking care of a quadriplegic that can't scratch his nose, whereas on the floor they usually could do some things for themselves.

Later in the interview, Adler compares her ICU and rehabilitation experiences:

Were there similarities in ICU and what you had been doing in rehab?

Yes, there are. There are an awful lot. To me, rehab was one of the best places in the world to learn good basic nursing care, because you are doing almost everything for the patient, but you are also trying to move them toward a level of independence as fast as you can. There is a lot of education. There is a lot of physical care. I am using those same principles with the bedside care in the ICUs now. It is really frustrating because nobody gives me credit for those three-four years that I did rehab nursing. As far as they are concerned I did not work those years. ICU is all that counts.

What made you burn out in rehab?

It was a staffing problem. There was a critical nursing staff shortage six years ago, and I was going to work, and on a routine basis, for 32 rehab patients. I would be the only rehab nurse, and I would have three agency nurses working with me. If anything went wrong, I was the one that was held to explain why this was allowed to happen, as if I could be in 32 places at once. I just could not stand that any longer because I could not give the level of care that I wanted to give. I was just—I felt that the hospital was being unbending, and they realized that we did not have enough nurses to take care of these patients, but they kept the beds full all of the time, and I finally got saturated to the point that I just could not take it and I just left.

You decided at that point to leave nursing?

Exactly.

Was that hard?

But I decided that this was just—I could not see where it was going to improve.

What was rewarding about working in rehab?

Because you saw people come in that really thought that they were not going to be able to do much of anything and by the time that they left—it is not the same goals that you would set for a normal floor patient—but they would be able to feed themselves with the assist devices, or a stroke patient would be able to start dressing himself. It was getting them through that process and getting them back on the road to going home again. It was really rewarding. I remember some really special times over there.

You established some very special contacts and relationships with the patients?

And they were long term. Some patients I took care of for three, four, or five months at a time, five days a week, and you really spend a lot of quality time with people.

Do nurses do things with those rehab patients that others didn't?

What nurses did was to pull together everything that all the other disciplines were doing because everybody else was looking at one section. The OT [occupational therapy] people were looking at hands, the PT [physical therapy] people were looking at feet and legs, and it was nursing that pulled it all together and said, "The reason that you have been doing all of this is so that you can learn to put a shirt on." We kind of integrated it for the patient. I think that we tend to be on the main conduit for the family a lot of times. We were a major family advocate, particularly with weekly patient care conferences that we had over there. I remember having one closed-head-injured patient [brain injury from trauma whose effects may not be visible as bruises or cuts, but behavioral] that every week I had to battle with the rest of the team about whether it was valid to keep him in the unit any longer or whether it was time to send him home. That was the one thing that I felt that nursing contributed to in that setting.

Barbara Bauer, thirty-seven, with over ten years of experience in an open heart surgery ICU since 1977, describes the rapid emergence of technology in that area, and the lack of clarity about roles and responsibilities. She begins by describing the rewards and frustrations of ICU:

What do you think is the most satisfying part of your work as a nurse in the ICU?

This is going to sound terrible, but the sicker a patient is, the more fun I've had. And the most satisfying is if I can get a super, super sick patient—and I mean we're talking balloon, ten drips, and bleeding at the same time—stable. I guess it's just going from absolute chaos when they come from the operating room to a point where everything is stable and at least on a level course rather than going downhill.

And knowing that you did this?

And knowing that I did it. Yeah. And you don't want to say by yourself, because you haven't done it by yourself. Obviously there's somebody sitting upstairs in the heavens that is sort of helping you a little bit, although the docs don't usually like to admit that. The docs have been there and then you've had your co-workers. But you like to say, "Hey, Mr. Smith is doing better because I was in there."

That you made a difference?

And I made a difference in his care. And every once in a while, in fact there was a note— One of the patients had a trach [tracheostomy] done last week at the bedside. And he had one of those tube holders in, which I hate. They're terrible to do good mouth care. But one of the physicians came in the next day after the trach and put a note in the chart. Wonderful mouth care done by nurse. And this was in the chart. Just a little comment that nurses have done wonderful mouth care. And I said, "Hey, that was me that did that wonderful mouth care after he had his trach." Okay, you don't have to have my name in there, but it sounds nice.

What about the most frustrating thing?

I think the reverse of getting that super sick patient on a stable course. It was eight years before I had a patient die on me, Jackie, in that intensive care unit. And I used to pride myself on that. You know that I could have a patient that they said wasn't going to last for fifteen minutes at seven o'clock in the morning and I would walk out at three P.M. in the afternoon and, granted, I might know that the patient might not be around in the morning because all signs indicated that he was moribund. But just to have a patient who's doing well, ready to go off to the floor you think, and then have a major infarct or a CVA in front of you. And knowing—I guess it's the frustration of something happening and knowing that there is absolutely nothing within your power— that feeling of powerlessness. You know, a patient who's bleeding— I remember one patient who was sitting up—well, not actually talking to us, she was intubated, but smiling, nodding, and we looked up at the monitor; and she was doing fine. We went to calibrate the monitor, and her eyes rolled back. Turned the monitor back on after we had recalibrated, and she was in electromechanical dissociation. And we never got her back. And no one knew what happened to her. She threw a clot to her conduction system or whatever. But this woman was fine. Why did this have to happen? And it was nothing that I did. I think I would probably feel worse if it were something that I had done.

Knowing you couldn't fix it—

I guess I'm to a point now where, you know, unless a drug is completely new on the market, I'm not afraid of giving the wrong concentration of drugs or anything like that. Those are the basics that are way behind me now. I can dial in and manage various drugs and know which ones are compatible and all this. Those are the minor things. But if it's something I cannot touch. And somebody up above said, "It's your time, Mrs. Smith"—that's the most frustrating thing for me.

What's the biggest change you've seen over the last ten years in nursing or in critical care in that unit? You mentioned earlier the nature of the patient population.

The nature of the patient population, but I think along with that you have to say the technology that has allowed that patient population to reach us, because ten years ago no one ever had a Swan [multilumen catheter that measures pressures in the heart and major blood vessels]. Everybody was done with central venous pressure [CVP] monitoring only, and that's probably why we didn't see seventy-five-year-old double valves with hypertension and diabetes. Now we've got a Swan, and we're doing cardiac outputs. We had the Swans and never knew how to do a cardiac output. I remember doing the first cardiac output with an anesthesiologist seven years ago. And then I think gradually just seeing the technology there, coming, but so much of it coming to us. It's like the physicians get their little toys. Swans were little toys for a while. And all of a sudden they become the domain of the nurse. Cardiac output—I remember the anesthesiologist doing the first one saying, "Barb, you want to try the second one?"

And then the third one—you're in charge.

And then the third one, well, it's yours. Onward we go. So, as the technology comes, we're expected to know about it. But it scares me in a way, because we're not electricians, you know. We're not surgeons. We're not anesthesiologists. They give us the technology, then, in a way, limit us. You know. We can't pull out the Swans. We used to be able to, and now the medical/legal aspects say not, in case it's wedged in the ventricle or the pulmonary artery, or something like that, you can't pull it out. So we've gotten in there and they sort of put restraints on us. Or a nurse comes from—well, we used to do all this— We used to pull out chest tubes—you know, we'd do this, that, and the other thing. No—can't do that here. Or the various— Or the opposite, a nurse coming to us saying, "Oh, we couldn't touch a Swan. I've never done a cardiac output before because that was the doctor's"—and so on.

Edith Hardeman describes the impact of technology on patients and nurses. She further reflects on the future of nursing as a consequence of the nature of the work and the media attention to the nursing shortage:

What's the biggest change in nursing you have seen?

Well, the biggest change, I think, is how we treat infarcts, how we treat patients going from the three-month stay in a medical bed to coming in, in the crisis of an acute infarct, getting TPA [tissue plasminogen activator, a drug that dissolves clots in coronary arteries], getting balloon angioplasty, and going home within the week. I think that is the biggest change. All that time we had to interact with patients, when we're sitting there giving them blood clots from leaving them in the bed too long. We went to this very high tech and very quick care. We've got to pack all the information into the patient at once, teaching everything in this high stress period of time, and I am seeing the acuity level go out of the roof because we are getting them turned over and getting them treated and out. It's kind of "treat 'em and street 'em." Whereas it wasn't before. We had time to get patients up to a certain level of wellness, while we had other patients that were pretty sick. Now I see us moving toward all intensive care in the acute care setting. Now people who are on the floor are the people who would have been in intensive care five or ten years ago. I don't see hospitals as places where someone can convalesce like we used to. We are in there being very aggressive, very quickly.

Is that a consequence of technology?

Well, I am sure it is. I think that people are better off for getting things treated quickly. I am not sure that their psychosocial needs are being met as well. I think physiologic needs are getting a bit better. I don't think their learning needs are enhanced or met any better. I think we are working harder to do it, to get it all in at once. I am not sure that we are doing a better overall job in nursing, doing what nurses do.

Sometimes we feel like traffic cops. You go here, you go there, we are gonna do this, or we are gonna do that first and then this, that kind of stuff, just directing traffic. Whereas before they would get this test done and a couple of days later they would get this test done and a couple of days later we would do something else. Meanwhile you would be preparing people all the way. Sometimes, now, we are running down the hall prepping [shaving the skin, cleansing it with disinfectant] somebody. I think that it is speeding up.

I am really worried that we are going to lose nursing, that nursing is going to become obsolete. Not because what we do is not valuable, in any way, shape, or form, but I don't know that we are going to get people that will be willing to do it. I think that all of the things that are going on with Oprah Winfrey and Sally Jessy Raphael and all these shows about the nursing shortage and all these nurses standing up and screaming about how terrible it is. I would not want to be a nurse if I were in high school and I saw that. I would not want to do that. How will we ever change a nursing shortage if we keep screaming about how bad it is? It doesn't make any sense to me. I think we have to do much more to promote nursing, what nursing is. One little test that I pull on people, "Can you name a famous nurse?" They say, "Yes, Florence Nightingale." "Can you name another famous nurse, maybe one who is alive?" They say, "No." Which means to me that the nurse is either the nurse that you had in the hospital, or the woman who lives down the street who goes to work at odd hours, or the person you see walking through the grocery aisles in her white uniform looking haggard with dirty shoes and with her hair a mess. We have to be careful of the image that we portray to other people, because we are nursing.

Hardeman continues to discuss the satisfaction and stresses of critical care nursing.

What is satisfying about CCU?

Well, I guess that I am odd or that I am getting older. I find what satisfies me in CCU is the same thing that satisfies me on the step-down floor—that is the patient contact. In my current position I don't get as much. I get involved in the really unusual situations rather than the average day-to-day. I ended up working Monday evening because we were very short on staff. I worked on the floor, and I haven't worked on the floor since my orientation. I was just running around and having a wonderful time. I had five patients that talked back to me. I love cardiacs. They talk back. I know people who say, in surgical intensive care, when they can talk to you it's time to move them out. I would hate that. I love talking with people. I talked with the five patients that I had that evening running from room to room doing patient teaching, getting them ready for cardiac cath in the morning, getting them ready for other tests the next day. That was fun. It's just fun to talk to people to get them to know that it is human to make a difference and go back the next day and ask, "How was your cardiac cath? Did you find it hard to lie flat for four hours? Did you feel the hot flash? How did you feel during the thing? Did you watch the test?" Having them give you good information back and then you can say, "I got through."

What is frustrating about nursing?

Not having time to do that.

Why do nurses leave nursing?

I think there are several different kinds of nurses. I think there are real nurses and I think there are appliance nurses. Have you ever heard that term? When the refrigerator goes out, they go back to work long enough to buy a new one and then they quit work. There are some real nurses and then there are some appliance nurses who just work when they have to. I think nurses, real nurses, leave nursing when there is too much conflict, when they are trying so hard—I think as a group we are pretty much perfectionists. Conflict occurs when you are trying so hard to be so perfect, and you find yourself in a situation where you can't do everything for a patient. Nurses leave because they get frustrated because they can't do all that they see themselves wanting to do. So they get out and do home health or get into something less stressful.

What has been the most stressful for you?

Well, I think probably that I had my own hardest time in dealing with the issue of dealing with abortion. Thank God I got out of OB [obstetrics] before they ever did anything like that. I worked on the third-floor CCU and around on the other end is the OB Department, and they were doing second trimester abortions, salting out. My friend came in one day and she was telling me that they did this saline abortion and the baby was born alive and immediately they started trying to resuscitate it. They worked on it forever trying to save it. I said, "Don't you have a problem with that? First you are trying to kill it and now you are trying to save it." Wait a minute, somewhere in here there is something wrong. It either is or it isn't. It can't be this way and when it doesn't work then we go the other way with it. That's when I started to define for myself what I felt I could live with. I support anybody's right to have one, a safe one. I could never do it, because I could never say that what was alive wasn't worth keeping until it was born alive, that then it was worth keeping. It didn't compute. I would never have gone back to OB/GYN services doing a lot of that because I couldn't face that conflict. I think a lot of critical care nurses get really really fried when they have to deal day in and day out with people who are getting treatments that they don't feel like are in their best interest in the long run. Things that save them, but for what? I do a lot of thinking about that.

How do you face it?

I think the way we all cope with these stresses is that we have to talk with each other. It is very difficult to talk to an outsider about it. You have to train somebody before they can understand what it is you are even talking about, the horrors of the decisions that you have to make and the things that you have to do. You just can't tell people.

We have to be able to talk among ourselves and support ourselves. We have to support each other, and I think psychiatric counseling has helped me out a lot to deal with how I felt about things and some of the ethical things. I think the whole issue of AIDS patients right now is horrendous. It is going to be awful. We have been talking the last couple of days about the plan to put an AIDS hospice in our hospital. I was thinking, "Who the hell would work there?" Somebody will. I wouldn't. We were trying to figure out who would do that kind of work. Somebody will, but it won't be me. I just couldn't take that kind of stress and strain every day of watching people die every day of that disease. Totally incurable. There are people who worked in polio hospitals and people who worked in TB hospitals. There will be people who will work in AIDS hospitals. My God. That would be so hard.

The terminal nature of the disease is the hardest part?

That and the population that you are dealing with. The average age is 36 to 38, the ones that I have taken care of. I have taken care of a lot of them, sitting in their room and them saying, "I want you to give so and so the picture over the fireplace and so and so the vase." You are in there dealing with that, and you are also dealing with the fact that he has put out nine liters of stool in sixteen hours. One liter, I am quite sure, went down from my waist all the way down my leg and into my shoe, because he had explosive diarrhea, and God, it was right there, and you say, "Just take me to the gas chamber, right now." I went in and I washed my leg off and washed my shoe out, and when I got home I just took everything off and dropped it. And I guess that I have not had this real fear of transmission to me. You are standing there, and I had worked a double shift with this guy. He has given you his last will and testament, and you are dealing with his lover, and you are dealing with his family members. He is telling you what it's like, and he has finally gone to sleep, and it's two or three in the morning, and you are exhausted. You have dumped untold amount of stool already, and he's got to get up, and he stands up, Mr. 1.9 potassium [1.9 milliequivalents per liter; 3.5–5.0 is a normal range; lower or higher values can be life-threatening because of the effect on cardiac muscle], and you worry about his heart, and he is weak, and he blows it all over you, and you say to yourself, "Do I have to do this? Is this what I have to do in order to make a living?" And the answer is no, you don't do this in order to make a living. You do this because of some other need. It may not be quite sane, but you don't need to do this to make a living. You do this because it is such a privilege to make such a difference in the lives of other people. Nurses have access to people the ways that nobody else does. At a cost. We pay a lot to do it.

Finally, Hardeman describes the satisfaction of allowing a "no code" (do not resuscitate) patient to die peacefully in an ICU setting:

Well, I remember the first time I ever let anybody die. I had a patient who was a "no code," and they were in critical care, and you sort of watched them fibrillate away. I remember feeling very guilty, because I knew there was some intervention that I could do under normal circumstances that would stop that process right then. It was a funny feeling sitting there watching somebody go and know that they were going. It isn't like finding somebody dead in the bed—it's there they go. This patient had liver cancer. His family was in the room and he was only about 38 years old. He was a young guy. I knew he was going to die, but apparently my staff did not. They had opened this unit with new graduates. Practically everybody had been out of school for two years, and they were all just holy terrors. Anyway, it seemed obvious to me that the man was going to die and he was a "no code." I was in there at about three o'clock in the morning and I said, "There he goes." He blocked down and there was a P wave, and then there was another P wave, and then a QRS [P, QRS, and T waves, as shown on an EKG or monitor screen, represent phases of the heart cycle], but it was bizarre in shape, and then another P wave. The staff was so upset and angry with me because I didn't go running into the room, because I didn't go immediately and tell the family, "There he goes." They were sitting in the room laughing at the time. I looked at them and said, "Isn't it better to go out of this world hearing the laughter of your family members than it is to hear, 'Oh shit, there he goes'?" They didn't understand. They didn't see that peace—we weren't going to do anything to change it. We weren't going to go into the room and make it better or easier. The family was in the room. They didn't see that.

I think I remember most clearly probably my first really critical patient. It was before we had intensive care and it was right after Aramine [a potent drug to elevate blood pressure] came out, and now it is gone, right? But I had the patient on an Aramine drip. His blood pressure was down, and there was something wrong with him. I can't remember what it was, but he had some sort of problem. I don't think that he was mentally retarded, but he was not quite right. I had worked with him all afternoon, and I had gotten his blood pressure up and stabilized on the Aramine, and this was out on a regular med-surg floor that had one RN for fifty patients. I went to that RN and said, "This is what I have done and I have gotten his blood pressure up and done all this," and I had stars in my eyes and she said, "You know he would be better off dead." I went to my instructor in tears and said, "How could she say that anybody would be better off dead?" I think about her sometimes. I still haven't said that anybody would be better off dead, because it stuck with me so long that nobody could be better off dead. But I think about it sometimes and I think, "Well, I have a bit more perspective." Not to say that in that situation she was right, because I don't think she was, but sometimes when I am looking at my patients and I don't know whether this is right. I don't know how far we should go with our technology. How much we should inflict on other people. Sometimes I think we do inflict too much just because it's there. The stuff just happens because it's there. And the decisions come later—or they don't.

Emily Vereen discusses the negative impact of technology on nursing care and nurse-patient interactions. She also touches on the ebbs and flows of her passion for nursing—the rewards and the fatigue.

The weariness is coming. It is nursing, it's not cancer. It is coming to grips with the fact that I no longer have the passion for nursing. It is almost like dying or losing a loved one. It is a mourning. Like there isn't very much more to learn, once you can do the bed pans and the injections and the medicine. It's like starting off making the beds. First you make the bed until it is perfect. The silly thing [instructor] comes in there and pops it to see how much resilience is on the bed and then you master that. Then you go and master the diet, you master the diabetic's diet. Then you master the injections. Then you master the pills, then you master the pumps, and you get new toys and trinkets all the time. When you have done all of those, it is kind of like over for me. I don't know if that has to do with nursing burnout, but what else is there to do?

What was appealing about nursing all that time?

Patients. It has been patients as well as things, because I am a things person. First off it was the drive to take care of the patients, and I think that is the only thing that still holds me. The machinery, really I think that the machinery takes away a lot. We were talking about this the other day. You have a probe here and a monitor here, and it tends to reduce the amount of tactile stimuli that you give the patient. You can walk to the foot of the bed and know everything that you need to know. You don't have to touch the patient. Sometimes I find people not even bothering to talk to the patient because he is intubated and he doesn't really respond, so guess what—neither does the nurse. She stands there. She looks, she reads, she thumps, and really, does she ever say, "It is going to be okay. It's Wednesday. It is a bright and sunny day. I wore a coat this morning. It is cold outside, but tomorrow is going to be warm"? We don't say anything to them. We will stand there and talk about their PO2 [blood oxygen levels] increase. We just don't talk to the patient. We talk about the patient and the machinery and I think that we—

I have seen you talk to patients.

I love to do that because oncology is that type of nursing. That is the passion that makes you want to take care and embrace that family and hold them and talk to them and talk to that dying person and let them know that you care and let them know that you give a hoot in a world that is so fast and even the physicians don't talk to the patients. When they come in, it's "are you feeling okay? Can I get you anything? Fine, well, we will see you tomorrow." Well, you may not see them tomorrow, and they are left with 10,000 questions, and usually, because the patient is so intimidated by the doctor, they don't want to take up his time because he is a valuable person to somebody else or my questions really aren't significant. So who else is left to embrace this person but the nurse. I love my patients. I cry. I am about to cry now when I think of all the people that I have lost, and I have lost some wonderful people, some ugly people, some nasty people. That is the passion for nursing. But I am too tired to do that any more. I don't want to do that any more. Maybe in five years I will have the same passion to do that again, I don't know.

Pat Dalton, thirty-one, a nurse with ten years of medical-surgical ICU experience in Florida, Indiana, and Georgia, beginning in 1977, now works in an urban trauma unit. She discusses the impact of technology on nursing care:

How does the use of increasingly complex technology influence the use of nursing time?

Well, I think it influences two aspects—it can either help nurses better utilize their time by freeing it up—cause you don't have to—you know you've got that visual. I don't have to go take my blood pressure with a cuff every time. I can watch my A line [arterial line], and it's quicker for me to glance at my monitor than to go listen, and I can still be doing something else. But again the time it takes to set up equipment, to troubleshoot equipment, to change lines, that kind of thing certainly takes away from nursing time. I think this equipment is here to stay, and we have just got to accept that, and we've got to learn how to make it benefit us and make it so that it does help us, whether it be through finding that right product that is helpful to us or to find the company that can make the right equipment and can back up their claims. That can be helpful to us.

How has technology influenced the environment in the ICU?

Well, for the patients it's got to be awful. I think it contributes an awful lot to our sensory overload in the unit. I mean the continual beeps and alarms and all that kind of stuff—you know that's certainly detrimental. It also clutters up your room. Sometimes it's hard to get to the patient through all the equipment. But, of course, the expense of it too. Sometimes I wonder if that's really justified.

Margie Goodrum, thirty-two, is a cardiology nurse with twelve years of diverse clinical experiences in rural and urban hospitals, beginning in 1975. She describes her perceptions of the impact of technology on resource allocation and the stresses on nurses in contemporary critical care units:

What is stressful about ethical dilemmas?

The most serious, I guess, is all the "no codes" that we deal with and, along with that, how aggressive to be with therapy. Medications are very expensive and, even before you get to the point when you make someone a "no code," if something happens to them, there is all this treatment. Sometimes I want to stop doing all this very expensive therapy that nobody thinks is going to do any good anyway. When we've got them on eight drips and they are doing all these scans and I'm thinking, "What are they going to do with all this information?" Giving them transfusions all the time. Blood, to me, is a pretty scarce resource and I would not hold it back from anybody who needs it, but I question, sometimes, the people we transfuse. The fact that you have so many groups to deal with, when it is the attending physician that has to make the decisions. The consultant physicians are the ones that have been doing every-thing because somebody asked them to and they may feel like that they ought to back off now. I had a surgeon tell me, "What we ought to do with this lady is turn off all of her drips and give her morphine. I am not going to open her back up. I don't want to know. I am not going to do any more scans on her belly because I know that she has more ischemic [very low oxygen level in tissue, which results in tissue death] bowel and I am not about to take her back to surgery. It would probably be financially lucrative, but it is an unethical thing to do. We ought to turn everything off and give her morphine." You know we couldn't because he could not make that decision. He was a consultant. Other ethical dilemmas are when is therapy appropriate or when is something the appropriate therapy? We still get people that I feel are inappropriate admis-sions who have tests done that are unnecessary. Who get very expensive hospitalizations for no good reason. Another ethical dilemma is when you can't get a physician to respond to something.

Does the existence of technology in the broadest sense deter-mine the kind of care someone gets sometimes? You talked about treatments being done just because they are there.

Yes, just because we are able to do something, then people automatically do it instead of evaluating whether or not we should do it. I always felt like our ability to do things has far outstripped our ability to decide when it is appropri-ate to do it.

How are these decisions made?

They are usually made by the physicians. They control the technology. They are the ones that order the medications and the technology. They are the ones that send people for scans. They are the gatekeepers to health care. They are the ones that admit patients to hospitals, and they are the ones that discharge patients from hospitals. They are the sources of revenue and the patients are their source of revenue. When somebody is in an ICU, I would think they get more money. With that kind of admission, I think that sometimes they do abuse the technology. Some do and some don't. Some are very good about saying, "Just because I could do it, would it give me any information that I can't get any other way? Do I really need to do this?" Sometimes people have a favorite scanner, so they scan everybody.

Why do nurses leave nursing? You don't see any sixty-year-old ICU nurses around, do you?

No, you don't. I think, first, because it does require a level of autonomy and responsibility that some nurses don't want. If you did not grow up with that, many times you get out. It gets to be very fast-paced and very intense and under the gun a lot of times, and sometimes people don't want that. I think a lot of times it requires a nurse who is younger and more assertive, who has been educated to think for herself and to recognize that what she does is not just based on what a physician tells her to do but that she has to make her own decisions. It is also hard physical work. You are turning and moving around a lot of very heavy people. You are on your feet and it is physically demanding. It is also mentally demanding. There is a lot of new technology, and if you don't know anything about it, it can be very frightening. It gets introduced, and if you get scared every time something new is introduced, you are not going to stay in the intensive care unit. That is where things get done. That is where the new technology comes in first.

Technology was perceived with ambivalence by most of the nurses interviewed. It made possible successful outcomes for older and sicker patients, but was seen as expensive and time-consuming and as often inappropriately used. Time was less available to nurses for teaching patients about their illnesses or even preparing patients for specific procedures in the most fundamental way, such as letting them know what to expect. Technology and fast-paced change compressed time, and the human dimensions of the environment and interpersonal exchange were often diminished. Further, roles were often unclear as technology was introduced and implemented. The existence of technology rather than decisions based on individual need often seemed to dictate its use. Competency and quality assurance with regard to technology both were assumed by nursing, but often very rapidly and with little time for preparation. Finally, technology was seen as stressful, because of complexity, rapid change, the demand for autonomy and responsibility with minimal authority for decision-making, and the general perception that technology often inflicts pain and unnecessarily prolonged suffering on patients when the timing of decision-making is awry.

Carla Olson, who was quoted earlier in this chapter, describes the impact of new technology on nurses. Her discussion epitomizes many of the issues related to the stress of technology that have been discussed, including rapid change, dealing with the unexpected, and the stress of the nurse preparing herself to be competent with new changes:

What about technology in the coronary care unit? It seems here to stay, and it's gotten more and more complex.

It feels like it couldn't possibly grow any more, but I know that it will. I'm sure that we're going to have to have automatic devices that adjust drug dosage according to changes in hemodynamic pressures and heart rate. We're going to have devices that measure, non-invasively, those things that we're now measuring invasively. I'm sure that we will have things on the outside of the body that measure cardiac output or something of that sort that don't require internal catheters, so maybe what's going to happen next is less invasive, but getting the same sorts of data.

More complex machines?

Oh, yes, definitely, more stuff, no question about that.

Do you think it has generally enhanced care?

Oh yeah, in terms of people living longer and surviving the infarct in a better way, oh yeah, no question about it.

Are there ways in which the technology inhibits care?

It doesn't inhibit physical survival. I think it may impair the emotional process of adjusting to things because there isn't as much time for the nurse to spend with you and let you know what's happening, but I'm sure it improves physical survival. And I wouldn't want to go back to not having it.

What about the challenge of preparing nurses to use it?

It's a challenge. If I don't get any help, I can't do it any more, not well and that's the honest to God truth. I can't be in a position of knowing that they need to know something and not having any resources with which to teach it to them. I don't fear the new technology, I just—looking back on it in my career I know that I didn't have any real way to really estimate the impact that it will all be new, and it will all be a shock—each thing that comes along. You just wouldn't believe it. You know, like the pill electrode, I enjoyed sharing that with the nurses, staff nurses, 'cause they would just laugh or they would look at you like—

The what?

The pill electrode, to get esophageal EKGs. Get big P waves, so you can tell subtle things about arrhythmias. You swallow this thing. It's a little wire and it has a monitoring thing on the end of it and it's in a pill. You put a gelatin capsule around it and you swallow it down to a certain level. They tape it to your mouth and hook it to your EKG machine, so the next time you have your tachycardia, you flip it on and you get an EKG from that wire to give you the business of P waves that are bigger than you traditionally get from outside EKGs. When I tried to share that with them, the shock and surprise and utter disbelief in their faces that they have for it just reinforces my own experience of each new thing, because I usually go through something like that too. You can't be serious—trying to decide if it's a joke or if it's really the next most wonderful thing. It's just very hard to tell because you are always on the cutting edge of thinking this is bizarre or this is really wonderful. [In 1994, esophageal EKG is an accepted standard in cardiac use.]

You are serious?

Very serious. That's exactly what they said, and then when they get over the idea of it, "Well, let me swallow one of these and let's see if it works." Well, it's just like a pill. Unless you gag with a pill, I don't think so, because the wire is extremely thread-like. But there is something new all the time, and everything you can think of can either be a joke or it could be the next most wonderful thing. Hard to say. And I don't remember it being like that early on. That seems to be more of the norm now. Well, we are always playing catch-up. The technology comes. You learn to use it and find out that you can't do it with the resources you've got, so you add more resources. No one can tell until the technology really comes what the demands will be.

The traditional nursing characteristics of caring, skill, and continual presence were augmented by a new aggressiveness as critical care settings became increasingly complex during the 1970s, 1980s, and 1990s. The nursing role was greatly amplified as nurses assumed responsibility for increasing numbers of technical skills. Technology influenced the practices of physicians and others in many medical and surgical specialties, for example, heart surgery in adults and children, renal dialysis, trauma care, and infectious disease. However, the technology at the bedside inevitably became the on-going responsibility of the nurse, often with very little anticipation or time for preparation. The various technologies, for example, ventilators, pulmonary artery catheters, cardiac, respiratory, and intracranial monitors, drug infusion pumps for almost any type of drug (narcotics, chemotherapeutics, vasopressors, vasoconstrictors, antiarrhythmics, metabolic support, and antibiotics), feeding tubes, and drainage devices (from the bladder, bowel, wounds, or chest cavity) — became routine patient care management strategies for the nurse at the bedside. Many support services emerged at this time to handle many of the technical aspects of one specialty, for example, renal dialysis technicians, anesthesia technicians, cardiopulmonary bypass technicians, and laboratory technicians. At this same time physician assistants emerged in a technical support role with physicians, and specialties in respiratory therapy and physical therapy began to develop. Nursing continued its traditional role of comprehensive patient care, perhaps in a medical or surgical specialty, while incorporating technology as it appeared at the bedside.

Providing adequate nurse staffing in hospitals, both in terms of quality of skill level and quantity, continued to be a problem. Two factors that influenced this issue were the insurance reimbursement systems by which hospitals receive operating costs and the organization of nursing services in hospital settings. Nurses are employed by hospitals. They do not bill patients for services. Nursing care, like housekeeping or dietary services, is included as a patient charge in the daily room rate. While recent efforts to "cost out" nursing services in hospitals and to obtain third-party reimbursement for nurses in independent roles have had some success with several insurance carriers and in several states, these cases remain in the minority. Many of the nurses interviewed identified inadequate staffing as a major stressor in critical care settings. These perceptions are consistent with the findings in the studies of nursing stress cited in Chapter 1 (e.g., Bailey, Walker, and Madsen, 1980; Jacobson, 1978; Strauss, 1968). Nurses generally identified hospital and nursing administrations as unresponsive to the highly stressful problems of understaffing or inflexible scheduling. Administrative reluctance to provide incentives to retain nurses, to increase nurse staffing, or to close hospital beds if necessary to provide safe nurse-patient ratios have, according to the nurses interviewed for this study, often resulted in attrition of nurses from staff nurse positions in hospitals.

Nurses continued to value their personal involvement with patients and their families, even as the demand for increasingly complex skill acquisition increased. Nurses described the conflicts inherent in these interactions. The primary motivation for patient involvement for the nurses interviewed seemed to be making a difference in the lives of patients in crisis. Nurses were willing to assume responsibility for very intense commitment to patients and families, but nurses acknowledged great frustration when patients were caught up in crises of indecision about the use of technology. Nurses described situations where the existence of technology dictated its use. Margie Goodrum, for example, stated, "Our ability to do things has far outstripped our ability to decide when it is appropriate to do it."

Nurses embraced the technology and became proficient in it. Indeed, the nurse became the major treatment modality at the bedside. However, nursing incorporated that skill level into traditional roles. While nurses learned to generate and use the increased amounts of data available for patient care and appreciated the positive outcomes for patients, many conflicts emerged in the care setting as a result of high technology. Decision-making about the uses of technology and the increased data that were available remains a problem at many levels. Time is compressed with many new technologies. Patients, nurses, and physicians once had weeks or, at least, days to incorporate data and change, to teach, learn, and prepare for a procedure or technique. At present decisions often have to be made instantaneously. Technology is relentless and demanding. Carla Olson said, "Well, we are always playing catch-up. There is something new all the time and everything you hear of can either be a joke or the next most wonderful thing."

Finally, when technology is backed by faulty decision making, the nurses viewed it as causing inhumanity and unnecessary suffering. While critical care nurses are not alone in dealing with these conflicts, the continual presence of nurses at the bedside and their particular combination of caring and skill make the model of critical care nursing unique.

3. The Art and the Science of Nursing Care: The Nurse and the Critically Ill Patient

The practicing nurse is almost invisible in the nursing literature. Case studies appear from time to time that reflect the intimacy of the nurse-patient relationship. These often relate the extraordinary experiences of nurses with, for example, dying patients, patients waiting for transplant, or children with leukemia. While the views of nursing's practice, education, and labor management leaders are well known, the evaluation of clinical practice has received less attention. For example, the literature may describe appropriate clinical management of a patient having heart surgery, but reveal nothing about the personal experiences of the nurses and patients during the actual caretaking. The stories of physicians and their patients have been more often told. The writings of Lewis Thomas (1983) and William Carlos Williams (1932) provide many examples of the range of human emotions and experiences in the medical care of patients.

The critical care nurses interviewed for this study spoke openly and often passionately about their beliefs and commitments about nursing and the rewards and frustrations of patient care. This chapter provides a forum for those nurses to speak about their perceptions of the essence of nursing practice. Many factors contribute to the nurses' perceptions about themselves and their practice. Several of these that have particular impact on the practice setting were selected for discussion: the roles that nurses assume; the values that permeate nursing education and practice; the accepted model of decision making in nursing; the ways that nursing has been defined by nursing leaders and others (because of the influence these definitions have on the formation of a professional self-image); and, finally, a research study examining clinical nursing practice from the perspective of practicing nurses.

Various disciplines have described the role of the nurse in critical care settings in relation to the medical, nursing, administrative, legal, historical, ethical, and even architectural dimensions of critical care. The nurse has been described as coordinator of patient care, collaborator with physicians and all other health team members, and promoter of activities to help the patient regain or maintain health (Kenner, Guzzetta, and Dossey, 1985: 4–5). Nursing functions in critical care have been defined by legal experts as including "interpretive and anticipatory functions of the nurse involving decision making and action with regard to a patient in biophysical and/or psychological crisis, close monitoring of patients in life-threatening situations . . . and rendering of life supporting treatment to patients who could not otherwise monitor the functional mechanisms underlying the life processes. The nurse must focus time and attention on mechanical aspects of treatment, anticipate subtle changes in patient status, and make quick decisions in emergency situations" (Garlo, 1984: 242–243).

Nursing roles have been described in a variety of contexts, but generally five roles are highlighted: practitioner, educator, consultant, researcher, and manager. Nurses also have been described as coordinators of care and as change agents. These roles have been consistent in the literature since the 1950s, regardless of the actual job title or setting (AACN Position Statement, 1987; Douglass and Bevis, 1983; Marriner, 1979; Menard, 1987).

Several concepts and values that have persisted in nursing education, nursing practice, and the nursing literature provide a conceptual framework for nursing practice. Patients are human beings with worth, dignity, and basic human needs that must be met. When these needs are not met, health problems or crises occur that require intervention by another person until the individual can resume responsibility for him- or herself. The patient has a right to quality health and nursing care delivered with concern, compassion, and competence. Increasingly, competent acute care or illness care is seen as a partial step toward wellness, prevention, and restoration. The therapeutic nurse-patient relationship is seen as a tangible and valid mechanism for healing. All behavior is meaningful, and individuals cope with crisis in proportion to their perceptions and resources (Harmer and Henderson, 1955; Hudak, Gallo, and Lohr, 1990; Kinney, Packa, and Dunbar, 1993; Moorhouse, Geissler, and Doenges, 1987).

Nursing as a process is recognized by various legal, professional, and accrediting bodies. The *Standards of Clinical Nursing Practice* set by the American Nurses' Association (1973) used nursing process as a framework as did the *Standards for Nursing Care of the Critically Ill* of the American Association of Critical Care Nurses (AACN) (Sanford and Disch, 1989).

The legal definition of nursing in most states includes a reference to nursing process (Georgia Board of Nursing, 1990: 3). Further, state boards of nursing require knowledge of nursing process for licensing by examination (Kinney, Packa, and Dunbar, 1993). The steps of the nursing process are derived from the scientific method. They include assessment (systematic collection of data relating to patients and their problems), problem identification (analysis and interpretation of data), planning (choice of solutions), implementation (putting the plan into action), and evaluation (assessing the effectiveness of the plan and changing the plan as indicated by current needs) (Hudak, Gallo, and Lohr, 1990; Kinney, Packa, and Dunbar, 1993; Moorhouse, Geissler, and Doenges, 1987). Nursing process is also a standard required by the Joint Commission on Accreditation of Healthcare Organizations: "Individualized, goal-directed nursing care is provided to patients through the use of the nursing process" (*AMH,* 1992: 79–80).

While nursing process became formalized as the appropriate model of decision making, other models have been proposed. The role of intuition and creative problem solving in nursing care was explored by Benner (1984). This model will be presented later in this chapter.

Implicitly, critical care nursing incorporates all the generally understood and accepted definitions and functions of nursing practice. The founder of modern nursing, Florence Nightingale, proposed the following definition in 1859. Nursing is "to have charge of the personal health of somebody . . . and what nursing has to do . . . is to put the patient in the best condition for nature to act upon him" (Nightingale, 1859).

Jane Van de Vrede was a nursing leader in the early twentieth century who was instrumental in setting practice and education standards in Georgia. While addressing the role of the public health nurse in 1921, when the focus of nursing was primarily private duty, public health, or Red Cross nursing, she proposed the following definition of nursing: "Prevention of illness and disability . . . is the unique function of the public health nurse, because of the acceptance of the nurse by the population, and the ability of the nurse to teach prevention . . . with the least presumptuousness and fear of being misunderstood. To this phase of health work, the nurse can make the greatest contribution" (Van de Vrede, 1921).

The anthropologist Margaret Mead, addressing a national nursing conference in 1956, made the following observation: "I have tried to identify this thing that everybody who is a nurse does, and how the service you give to our society could be phrased. It seems to me that you protect the vulnerable, that you protect all those who are or could be in danger, in any kind of danger — from illness, from strain, from shock, from fatigue, from sorrow, from grief; that every spot in this society where there are those who are in danger and who need continuous concern, this is the place where you might function" (Mead, 1956). This definition seems an almost prophetic vision of the roles and relationships that exist between critical care nurses and very ill, dependent patients in the highly technical, rapidly changing contemporary critical care unit. Never, in the history of modern nursing, have patients been so vulnerable, so much in danger and in need of continuous concern.

Virginia Henderson, a nursing leader and educator, first proposed her definition of nursing in the 1940s. This widely accepted definition likely influenced the self-concept of generations of nurses in the United States to the present. "Nursing is . . . assisting the individual, sick or well, in the performance of those activities contributing to health or its recovery (or to a peaceful death) that he would perform unaided if he had the necessary strength, will, or knowledge. And to do this in such a way as to help him gain independence as rapidly as possible" (Henderson, 1961: 42). She updated this definition in 1985: "The unique function of the nurse is to do for others what they would do for themselves if they had the strength, the will and the knowledge; and to do it in such a way that the recipient of the service acquires independence as soon as possible or an ability to cope with a health handicap, or to die with dignity when death is inevitable" (Henderson, 1985: 5). The subtle differences between the definitions reflect language changes, but also an assumption that nurses assist patients with activities related to self-care and coping with the outcomes of illness. The change may indicate areas of evolution and maturity in nursing and in Henderson herself during those years.

Georgia's Nurse Practice Act gives the following definition:

> Practice of nursing as a registered professional nurse means the performance for compensation of any act in the observation, care and counsel of the ill, injured, or infirm; and in the promotion and maintenance of health with individuals, groups, or both throughout the lifespan. It requires substantial knowledge of the humanities, natural sciences, social sciences, and nursing theory as a basis for assessment, nursing diagnosis, planning, intervention, and evaluation. It includes, but is not limited to, provision of nursing care; administration, supervision, evaluation, or any combination thereof, of nursing practice; teaching; counseling; the administration of medications and treatments, as prescribed by a physician practicing medicine in accordance with Article 2 of Chapter 34 of this title, or a dentist practicing dentistry in accor-

dance with Chapter II of this title, or a podiatrist practicing podiatry in accordance with Chapter 35 of this title. (Georgia Board of Nursing, 1990: 2–3)

The American Nurses' Association proposed the following definition of nursing in 1980: "Nursing is the diagnosis and treatment of human responses to actual or potential health problems" (American Nurses' Association, 1980: 9). In addressing the question "To what extent are popular definitions of nursing consistent with traditions and generally sanctioned social mission?" Rosella Schloffeldt (1987: 64–67) critiqued the ANA definition as ambiguous and lacking clear logic. She proposed, instead, the following: "Nursing is the appraisal and the enhancement of the health status, health assets, and health potential of human beings" (Schloffeldt, 1987: 67).

Definitions of nursing seem valuable to the extent that they direct values and attitudes or reflect them. The reflections of critical care nurses may forge new dimensions of self-appraisal. Patricia Benner conducted paired interviews with novice and expert nurses in order to "uncover the knowledge embedded in clinical nursing practice" (Benner, 1984: ix–xv). The interview data reveal the following domains of nursing practice: the helping role, the teaching-coaching function, diagnostic and monitoring functions, management of rapidly changing situations, administering and monitoring therapeutic interventions and regimes, monitoring and ensuring the quality of health care practices, and organizational and work role competencies. Benner's domains and the competencies for each domain are listed in Table 1 in order to form a framework for interpreting the interview material and case studies in this book and as a reference for the non-nurse reader to clarify the scope of nursing practice. These domains of nursing practice provide a clear descriptive framework for nursing practice and are consistent with the themes described by critical care nurses interviewed for this study.

Several themes predominated as critical care nurses spoke about nursing practice and their motivations, satisfactions, frustrations, and perceptions of their value. Almost universally, they expressed some type of commitment about self, nursing, and caretaking. Many spoke of nursing as a vocation and expressed a desire to make a difference in the lives and health outcomes of patients and their families. Even nurses who were more neutral about vocational commitments seemed heavily invested in nursing, patients, or the clinical situation. None of the nurses interviewed seemed

TABLE 1   Domains of Nursing Practice and Identified Competencies

---

The helping role

The healing relationship: creating a climate for and establishing a commitment to healing

Providing comfort measures and preserving personhood in the face of pain and extreme breakdown

Presencing: being with a patient

Maximizing the patient's participation and control in his or her own recovery

Interpreting kinds of pain and selecting appropriate strategies for pain management and control

Providing comfort and communication through touch

Providing emotional and informational support to patients' families

Guiding patients through emotional and developmental change

The teaching-coaching function

Timing: capturing a patient's readiness to learn

Assisting patients to integrate the implications of illness and recovery into their lifestyles

Eliciting and understanding the patient's interpretation of his illness

Providing an interpretation of the patient's condition and giving a rationale for procedures

The coaching function: making culturally avoided aspects of an illness approachable and understandable

The diagnostic and monitoring function

Detection and documentation of significant changes in patient's condition

Providing an early warning signal: anticipating breakdown and deterioration prior to explicit confirming diagnostic signs

Anticipating problems: future think

Understanding the patient's potential for wellness and for responding to various treatment strategies

Effective management of rapidly changing situations

Skilled performance in extreme life-threatening emergencies: rapid grasp of a problem

Contingency management: rapid matching of demands and resources in emergency situations

Identifying and managing a patient crisis until physician assistance is available

Administering and monitoring

Starting and maintaining intravenous therapy with minimal risk and complications

Administering medications accurately and safely

TABLE 1   (*Continued*)

Combating the hazards of immobility
Creating a wound-management strategy that fosters healing, comfort, and appropriate drainage

Monitoring and ensuring the quality of health care practices
Providing a backup system to ensure safe medical and nursing care
Assessing what can be safely omitted from or added to medical orders
Getting appropriate and timely responses from physicians

Organizational and work role
Coordinating, ordering, and meeting multiple patient needs and requests: setting
priorities
Building and maintaining a therapeutic team to provide optimum therapy
Coping with staff shortages and high turnover

Source: P. Benner, *From Novice to Expert: Excellence and Power in Clinical Nursing Practice*
(Menlo Park, CA: Addison-Wesley, 1984).

indifferent, negative, or impersonal about the nurse-patient interaction.
Nurses believed that they made a difference to patients through their
competence in the actual care that was delivered. Especially in critical care
settings, nurses made an impact through clinical management of the total
patient situation. Nurses accomplished this through coordination, competence, expert clinical judgment, and advocacy. Expert clinical judgment and
advocacy often involved anticipating subtle changes in patient status before
they occurred, acting on them appropriately, monitoring medical management, and initiating action to obtain competent medical care. The nurses
saw themselves as making the hospital system work for patients.

Nurses described a great deal of satisfaction from nurse-patient interaction, regardless of the setting. Nurses used the phrase "nurses take care of
patients" often. And "the only reason patients need to be in the hospital is
nursing care." One nurse described the challenge of "instant intimacy."
Nurses and patients, although strangers, may bond quickly when brought
together by the crisis of illness in a critical care environment. Nurses can
often humanize this situation of crisis, chaos, illness, and life and death
balances. Further, the process of investment of self seemed to humanize the
interaction for both the nurse, the patients, and those family or friends close
to them.

Lee Usher describes her views about the meaning and commitment
involved in critical care nursing:

I can just tell you the only thing you need to do is go and see those patients who are coming back from a heart transplant or coronary bypass or a valve replacement or anything, and they are lying there, and they are just as— as unconscious as they can be. They haven't recovered yet. And just watch the sensitivity and the caring and the look in those nurses' eyes and how they keep those patients warm. There are so many lines going in and out until I don't know how they know what line. But you can see the sensitivity and the feeling and the caring.

Where does that come from?

It comes from the individual person, I think. The kind of person that usually wants to be a nurse, and I think also—that's the spirit of nursing. And I think that nursing is a profession—it's a service profession, and the only reason for our existence is to be of service to society. Now there are lots of ways in which we can serve, but I believe so much of it is the—it's the embodiment of what nursing is all about and that's caring and nurturing and so forth, and it also—you have to learn a lot, so you have to have lots of knowledge and skills and so forth. But it's that caring.

Is that what's unique about nursing for you, the caring?

I think what is unique about nursing to me is that total kind of commitment to—and I'm not saying to be a martyr or that it's charitable or anything, but I think that is what is unique about nursing. That is what makes us so privileged. I used to think that we were—and I still think it—but that was when I was involved more with patients and families than I am now. But I used to feel like I was so privileged just to be a part of this experience in other people's lives, and I know that I have had more experiences in a week's time than some people have in a lifetime. And it's because of being a nurse and being involved with people. And I think that is extremely important that nursing is a noble profession and a noble calling, but I also think that we need to be recognized for it. It's not something that we aren't to be recognized for, and know that we just serve without pay or without recognition. I think that we have to have our professional status as a profession and as individuals and that we need to be properly compensated.

Lisa Fields's experiences have all been in hospitals, many of them in critical care. She is also an artist and has worked as a nurse while completing a degree in art and pursuing creative outlets. She speaks of the ways in which nursing has provided opportunities for meaningful human interchange in her life:

Actually, this is just an issue of mine, when I went to art school my teachers—they just made a comment that it did not look like my work, my outlook had anything to do with nursing. They would say surely you have experiences that you are emotionally involved with, that affect you. Why don't we see any of that? I think that what I have done is just wrapped myself so severely that I really did not know how to open up. That has been part of my goal in the past few years—to let the walls come down and let my emotions out. I would have to say in terms of my own personal growth, it has been—because of my experiences in intensive care with dying people just the way that has affected me and my understanding about the life process. So in that sense it has affected me because I felt very connected with the process that people go through being linked with illness, death, and recovery, whatever it is. In a way it seems like a lot of people in cultural art are really alone and isolated. I know that's what is expected in my state of being and I understand that. It just has made me feel very connected to what it is about to be human and to live here on earth and not in my head—just on a real day-to-day level, what it is like to be human. One of the things that seemed like an extra thing that I would never have thought about is one of the things that I really love about nursing, when people come to the hospital they are in a crisis situation, and that it is a crisis no matter what they come in for—that it creates a situation for them where I think that they are much more open and that there is someone there available to help them and they are just much more open emotionally than they normally would be on the street. Let's say if I met this person at a bank or something. Because of this crisis they are more vulnerable and open and I have this opportunity to interact with them. The shields are down. Their barriers are down and so my barriers are down and we can really connect with each other from a very heart-centered place. I have really experienced what I would perceive as true communication because it is not just words, it is really from the heart. That has also been my experience with healing in a hospital setting—it has been through that kind of open channel of communication. It is just a flow of energy between myself and the patient, and I feel like it has been not only a healing for the other person but one for me as well. You know because it is an openness to the true sense of who you are—In a way, it is a spiritual experience there too.

So there is a philosophy there too? Do you think that there is something unique about nursing that facilitates that?

Yes. I guess that it is possible to connect with people in that way outside of the hospital business. You know I had an experience when I was traveling, and

I met somebody on a train, somebody I was going to only see very briefly and have an extremely intimate connection with them—somebody I would never see again. In a way that is very much like that, but it is just kind of these unexpected places that you connect with people, but they seem to happen more frequently in hospitals. I think it is because the people—patients—are in crisis, and they are more open emotionally to receiving what is available to them, any help from any place, any support from anyone, because they are scared. So it is easy to come in and establish a rapport with a patient based on trust. And intuitively, if they think that they can trust you, they open up all kinds of things. Like I am going to be here and establishing that trust. I think that it is more available to nurses to make that kind of connection than physicians because nurses spend so many more hours with patients than doctors do. And, plus, you are nurturing, and nurturing concepts are sort of inherent to nursing more than anything else.

Fields describes her role with patients in the critical care setting:

Tell me about your patients. What needs do they have?

I would say that they have acute physical, medical, or surgical needs as well as emotional ones. The full range. A couple of patients that I can think of. One of them was a chronic GI [gastrointestinal] bleeder—gastric ulcer—and she looked pretty bad, had been unstable all day but not really. My involvement with her was just the continual assessment and also the emotional support of her husband, he was obviously very devoted and terrified. Also to her because she was scared. I think that is a lot of what the need is, is in doing the patient's care. By the time I had left she had started vomiting copious amounts of bright red blood and that was when we started calling the doctor, putting a tube down her and doing lavage and dealing with her vital signs at the same time she was stabilizing. What was her blood pressure doing, pumping fluid into her veins. Trying to give her husband some support. He was outside, but informing him and reassuring the patient, assisting the doctors, and trying to keep everything running smoothly. Making sure all the supplies were available. And keeping the drugs going.

What difference do you think that nurses make in an ICU setting?

They make a lot of difference, mainly because of their ability to assess. You know there are so many major problems that if they are caught right away you can avoid total disaster for a patient. Whereas, if the nurse isn't tuned in or perceptive or skilled or educated about assessment skills, when the small problems are the beginnings of big problems, a patient can go down the tubes too fast to be brought back.

Do nurses make independent decisions and assessments in ICU?

Very independent, more independent than on the floor. Especially in directing patient care, suggesting everything from treatments to medications to protocols and also being patient advocates at the same time. What is and isn't appropriate for a physician to prescribe not just in terms of what the patient's medical condition is but also what may or may not be necessary at that time. Whether an inappropriate test is going to be real expensive for the patient, that kind of thing. Especially in ICU the nurses are really the trouble shooters. They are the ones that see it first. They have to know what they are seeing and know that they are seeing something and call the doctor. The nurses I work with, the ICU nurses, are incredible in their ability to really see the forest and the trees. They can really pick up on things. They are sort of the integrated masters there, because in a way I even see that it really is not the doctors, it really is the nurses that pull it all together and tie it together in a pie. The doctor sort of fits into that pie, but it is the nurses that not only run the show behind the scene but through it all. They are just the fabric of the care of the patient that holds it together.

What do you think that nurses do that is most important?

I think that their most important function is a protective, promotive function. Protective in a sense that would involve assessing and protecting them from whatever is their illness inside of them. Also protecting them from succumbing to problems, problems that could arise either from poor care, poor management, or mismanagement. Also promoting their optimum level of health: teaching them, in terms of decreasing their possibilities of reoccurrence, or their residence in the hospitals, on whatever level that they can do that. I would also include in that the emotional support that nurses do promote that they [the patients] are not alone. I think it is like the way that fear can immobilize the immune system for one thing from stress, the stress of fear. One of the ways that nurses can really help people is to help them to mobilize their systems towards health, towards fighting whatever their diseases are or their problem is for being in the hospital. Teaching them emotional support against fear so that they have a sense of connectedness with a key human being. What I would imagine is a totally overwhelming environment, overwhelming in terms of its size and also its technology, especially in ICU. When I think about looking at it as an outsider, somebody that comes in for a cardiac cath, an outpatient who comes in for a cardiac cath and ends up with an evolving AMI [acute myocardial infarction], in a unit. I mean, what a nightmare! These monitors. They weren't prepared. They can't look out the window. They are on these uncomfortable little beds—just all of the equipment around them. Everybody is dressed in green. I think that one of the most appropriate things that a nurse can do in that environment is to be a human, since the patient doesn't expect that I am a human, but that I am a system. When you said to me, "what is the most important thing that nurses can do for a patient," what really popped into my mind was that they can be involved. It is the heart, the nurse's heart, really—the heart and the mind have to be flowing at the same time, but the heart has got to be there too. There was a nurse in report, and all you get is emotional data about the patient. Following her was a total nightmare. She never had anything done right. Drips would be off. Ventilators and alarms would be turned off. Medications would be wrong. It was like really the patient needs to get his medications, and the patient needs to have the right drip rates and the patient needs his food and IVs and skin care, and he also needs emotional support, but he really needs both of these. That is what nursing does. It combines the head and the heart, I think.

Fields goes on to speak about the meaning to her of working with dying patients and, finally, of her nursing care of a patient in pain:

You mentioned that nursing has been very positive to you. In what way?

By giving me exposure to people dying. I feel like that is a very rare treasure and a privilege most people never accomplish. Being able to see babies born and being able to see people die. I feel like it makes me feel very connected to myself and my human process. Experiencing what life is and being a human being. Sort of like television is to the general public: people getting off on other people having emotional crises as they do in hospitals. TV is the closest thing most people can experience about life and death. People who have problems go to certain places and professionals take care of them. But I feel, in a way, it is exhilarating to me, and what it has taught me I could not have learned anywhere else than being a nurse in a hospital. The experience that I have had, I have never heard anyone else talk about it. I have really experienced it within my body, this sort of acceleration of energy, and it feels like massive amounts of vibration and the frequency picks up so much I feel it inside my body. It is like when the pulse stops. Is there a blood pressure? And I look at the body and there is no life in the body. It is a good and a bad feeling. The life force is so full of energy that it is finally liberated. It is amazing—used to, when I would get a "no code," I would think that it was such a treat because I would be with that person when they died. It is such a personal thing and such a privilege.

I had a patient who was in her early thirties and had radical chest surgery and had some kind of chronic nerve damage. They could not alleviate the pain. When I came on they told me she had been getting Dilaudid [narcotic pain medicine] all night and she had been up all night. When I came on, I thought, okay, this is wrong and that is wrong—and I told her that I was going to change her bed. I got her into the chair and she was in a lot of pain. I gave her a bath, washed her back, and as I was washing her back, I was thinking that I did not know how to do this, but I was going to try something here. I had both my hands on her back and was rubbing her back and I really prayed and let myself be an open conduit and I just kept rubbing her back and focused my whole being on her. She started talking about her family, and how she has pain, and when she doesn't let her husband have any sex, he is angry, and all the rules, and he is angry because she isn't home to cook and take care of the kids, and that she was just so depressed, and he just could not accept her little boy, and on and on. Finally, she stopped talking and she slept for about four hours. Then she went to physical therapy and had a treatment. She did not have anything for pain the rest of the evening until about four in the afternoon and she started having pain again. After about an hour or so she was in bed, and she said that she wanted me to do the same thing that I had done that morning for her. I told her that I did not know if I could but I would try. A couple of the family members insisted on staying, an aunt or something. They were just real skeptical like, "What are you going to do to her?" I did not feel real comfortable with them staying. I just went through the same process of rubbing her back and talking to her and just really kind of being quiet, and she mentioned this, too. I walked out of the room with the two family members. One of them asked if I hypnotized all my patients without their consent. Well, she asked me to do the same thing that we had done this morning and that was it. They both looked really offended and angry. They did not understand what had happened, obviously, and they seemed very much out of control. I just let it go at that. It was a really interesting experience. "But don't you see she is not hurting any more?" It was really interesting to me the possibilities to explore and to be more careful with this kind of thing. It doesn't matter if the pain goes away, if it is an unconventional method, it isn't okay. The drugs are fine, but a back rub and relaxation are not okay.

Annie Kelly, thirty-six, a nurse for fifteen years, beginning in 1972, is a critical care nurse who has worked in hospitals and schools of nursing in

Pennsylvania and Georgia. She is currently working as a nurse and studying for a Ph.D. She describes a patient interaction in a suburban community hospital near Atlanta that provides an example of advocacy:

The last time that I worked there was a twenty-one-year-old that was from Michigan. He was down here working. His family was in Michigan and he is a subcontractor and has no insurance. He was living down here with his girl-friend's family. He was working on a roof and fell 35 feet. He fractured his pelvis and hand. He was very fortunate that he did not have head trauma, but he did have his head all banged up and was in intensive care. This was his first day there when I took care of him; then I worked two days in a row, so he was one of my patients those two days. I talked with him about himself. In report, I never got that he was down here by himself or that he was self-paid, or that he was living with his girlfriend's family. I found that out through talking with him when I did his assessment. He was very lucid and was very concerned about his hospital bill. He was planning on going to work a week after he got out of the hospital. When the orthopedic physician came in, I facilitated conversation between them by specifically saying, "Mr. So and So is particularly interested in when he can go back to work." The physician told him anywhere between twelve and fifteen weeks. Again, that is not conducive to his lifestyle because he can't live here by himself with no money. His dad died six months prior with cancer so this family—looking at the total family picture—had a lot of stress. His mother was on the phone wondering how her son was down here because she did not have money to fly down and see him.

This provides one example of facilitating and intervening on an ethical issue. The orthopedic fellow said he was going to send this cast man over to cast his hand, and the young fellow said, "Is that necessary?" and said that he was worried about it. The orthopedic fellow said, "Yes," because he was going to have to be up on crutches and when you are up on crutches he would need a cast on his hand so he could support himself and not put pressure on his hand. When the physician left I went back into the room, and he wanted to know how much that was going to cost, and I told him I was sure that it was going to cost at least a hundred bucks for him to come over and put the cast on. He said even if it cost fifty it was too much money, and he really did not want him to do it. I repeated that, and he agreed that was what he said. I went out and caught the doctor going down the hall and said, "Come on back. This patient needs to talk to you," and he said, "What about?" I told him that I thought that he did not want the cast on, and the doctor gave me a dirty look, like, "What have you been in there telling him?" He went back in, and the patient said, "I really do not want the cast on, because I am not going to be walking around that much anyway for the first couple of weeks, and I don't think that I need it. I am paying for this myself. Can't I just use the splint that you have on me now?" The physician—you could tell that his ego was quite irritated about the patient refusing treatment. The physician said, "That is fine, that is fine with me," and he said something to the patient, like, "Well, if you hurt yourself, don't go taking me to court." He left, and I checked his notes later—that the patient refused treatment, but he did not say why. I thought that was inappropriate. He should have looked and noticed that the patient was self-paying and could we use something else that would be less expensive for the patient. I found out later when I called PT (physical therapy), because he was supposed to learn how to do crutch walking, that PT said since he did fracture his hand they weren't going to give him the regular crutches anyhow. They were going to give him the kind where you put your whole forearm in anyhow. Whereas the physician thought that he was going to be putting pressure on his hand. So it all turned out okay. But it could have turned out nastier if I had not intervened in communicating the patient's needs. The patient would have been more anxious. He even told the doctor, "If they put the cast on, once I get home I am going to cut it off because I don't think that I need it." That is when I said we will just get him not to put it on. His mother called long distance, so we rolled him out in the bed and let him use the phone at the nurse's desk.

Was he in a body cast?

No, he was just on bed rest because his pelvic fracture was a vertical fracture and he just needed to be maintained on bed rest. It wasn't one that they would call an unstable fracture. He could get up and move around. We rolled him out and let him talk to his mom, and that was ironic because five years ago you would never allow that. I think that is another example of accommodating the patient's needs, not only in communicating with the family, but physicians too, and meeting his needs as an individual. There were his concerns of being self-paid and that he needed to get back to work as soon as possible. He is young—an older patient might have just told the doctor right then, "No way, you don't put a cast on my arm." Then again a younger patient as such, especially since his dad had just died in an intensive care unit six months ago, I am sure he had a lot of anxiety, being in an intensive care unit.

Margie Goodrum has worked both in a small, country hospital, where she was the only nurse for operating room, recovery room, intensive care, and emergency room, and, currently, in cardiology/CCU (coronary care unit) in a teaching hospital in Atlanta. She describes the impact that nurses have on patient care, especially documenting subtle changes, as well as a patient care situation where nurses personalized the care of a patient to help her with her dying:

What difference does the nurse make in an ICU setting?

A tremendous amount. It is the nurses who have a feel for what is going on with the patient and know what direction the patient is moving in, whether he is getting better, when it is not quantitative things. When you can't say, "Oh, his blood pressure has now stabilized at 120 over 80." It goes beyond that. They feel that during their time that they were with the patient that they made some changes and some progress. It is just a feeling that it was a positive thing and not a negative thing. There are nurses who are better at assessing, who catch things earlier, who recognize a trend before it becomes a change. Everybody can recognize a change, but it's the subtle things that they see early. It's following up on details. It's following up and making sure that everything gets done as it was supposed to have. Following up on—and deciding what's needed is—assessing them not according to protocol. I hate vital signs every fifteen minutes on the floor, because I think that it is taking away from the nurse her prerogative to assess what the patient needs. There have been times when I have stayed right beside a patient and assessed him constantly. There have been other times when I have known that it was okay to leave him for even as much as a couple of hours in the unit, because he is being monitored anyway. I can devote my attention to someone else and know that he will call me if he needs me. It's those kinds of things that you know as organization and being sure that things get done. It is a very important experience as a nurse.

Do all nurses do it?

No, I think it's not just a function of time, it's a function of time spent and also opening your mind up. Trying to learn. Some nurses just remember experiences. I think it's experience housed on experience, and you start seeing certain patterns and start putting things together. I think that you have to be open to that and have to supplement that with some basic knowledge and seek further knowledge. I think that experience has to be supplemented by knowledge and theory. You have to understand that if something occurs frequently in a certain condition or a certain type of patient then you need to know what is the basis for which this might occur. You might have some theoretical knowledge, and some scientific foundation on which to hang that. It takes both. It is not just a function of time. Some people have been there a long time and they still do not recognize patterns and individual responses.

What is it that nurses do that is most important?

I think, from the patient's perspective, it is a cross between being competent and caring. I think it is those two Cs. I think that they don't always recognize the things that we do, but they know who is competent. Even if they can't put words to it and say, "She recognized that," when they started feeling a little funny, the nurse was right there and she did something. She either reassured them or she gave them a medication, she did something. She told them this is what happened, this is why you feel this way, your blood pressure is fine. It is knowledge and caring, the two together. They may not know exactly what it is that we know, but I think particularly in a unit they see that a nurse doesn't get all flustered and say, "I don't know, maybe I'll call the doctor." I think that they recognize that you can say, "What is going on?" or "I don't know, that is hard to say."

You had mentioned earlier, before we started taping, about a particular patient that you had humanized an experience for.

That was a patient who was very frustrating for us. She was not a cardiac patient; she was thoracic and pulmonary service. She was a long-term ventilator patient, and she was very difficult to deal with. Her defense mechanism was denial, and she was one of these passive, health-rejecting people that needs help, but everything was rejected. I liked her, and I think most of us liked her as a person even though she frustrated the devil out of us. She was in the hospital from January until July. She was in our unit, ventilator-dependent from March until July. We were not a unit that likes long-term ventilator patients. We had a few but never anyone this long and never anyone that we tried so hard to wean, and she had a very high anxiety level. She rejected everything that we tried to do for her in some way. Very passive, and it was very frustrating because we had to realize that we could not be Jean's motivation. That we could not, me especially, find that magic phrase that would make Jean want to fight, want to work. Because every step of the way, weaning her, she resisted. It finally came to the point that we had a party for her. It came about because I was talking to her physician who had been taking care of her for a couple of days. We were talking about her chances of ever getting off the respirator. While she had made progress, it had been since March, and this was June or early July that she was still off the vent a total of six hours and on the vent for one hour, then back off the vent for six hours, and overnight she was on the ventilator. It had been a struggle with a lot of setbacks. I said that if she ever does get off that we were going to have a party because she told one of the nurses that she liked champagne and strawberries. He said that we should have the party at the halfway point and let's consider this the halfway point. I said if you will bring the champagne, we will bring the strawberries. Then we planned it further. The other thing she wanted was to see her dog. We even went through infectious disease control and had the dog clipped and bathed and brought it in, in a suitcase, with holes in it, into her room. We had champagne, strawberries, whipped cream, and balloons. I think it was more for the nurses than it was for Jean. She was just a very difficult patient, but we all liked her.

How old was she?

Fifty something, she was not that old. She had thoracic surgery for an empyema [lung abscess—infection], and even before she was ventilator-dependent, physical therapy had said that she was a patient that they could hardly get out of bed to ambulate her. They had been called in to help the nurses get her up and moving around. She was just a strange kind of person. She had a lot of setbacks. We had her where she was even walking some in the unit, and we would take her out of the unit, and we had said the next sunny day we were going to take her out to the courtyard. But it never came to that. She had some setbacks, and she decided that she did not want to do this and she did not want to live like this. She didn't see any hope. She communicated to her daughter that she was ready to die, and it was decided that we would let her do that. We gave her morphine, and she started going downhill, and basically what we did was keep her comfortable. She used to have severe anxiety attacks, and it wasn't anything physical, it was mental. She had a respiratory rate in the 60s and 70s and she would just wear herself out. The decision was made that we would not wean any more and that she was ready to die and we would let her die. We still have pictures of the party. The psychiatrist had staff conferences on her, and he was very helpful to the staff and was very encouraging about what we did. Because of the nurses' care of Jean her family asked that there be no flowers but that contributions be given to the hospital in honor of the nursing staff in CCU. It was really nice and it helped us. It was such a long thing. We rotated Jean among the staff because you could not deal with her for more than four or five days at a time, because we were trying to be her motivation. You can't be that for somebody, but that is what we do a lot of times.

Who takes care of nurses?

Sometimes nobody. We don't take good enough care of ourselves. But we tried with the staff conferences to express what we were feeling. I know our clinical coordinator talked to the psychiatrist a good bit, and she told him how important that it was that we need to know and we needed to get some feedback. That we were okay, and we were doing the best that anyone could do. She was so difficult, except for what she wanted to do, which was not much except lie in bed.

Denise Clements, introduced in the Introduction, describes the coordinator role of the ICU nurse and the caretaking that she believes patients expect:

I see the role of the nurse in ICU to be overseer of all the disciplines, patient advocate. My God, the patient needs nursing. And you know, who's going to take care of the poor sucker in the bed? It's the ICU nurse. Who's going to look over what everybody else is doing? It's the ICU nurse. I mean you should see it in the code, Jackie. I'm sure you have. It's like thirteen people standing around talking about what needs to be done, and three people doing the work and all the three are the nurses. Just like at a construction site on the road. We actually deliver the care. And we can do the chest physical therapy, and we can do the pulmonary toilet; we can do all of those things. I think there's a need for some more specialization and I don't have a problem with that, but I would like—I believe that nurses—the nurse's role is to be the planner, the overseer, the evaluator over all of what's going on with the patient, and truly it falls to nursing to interpret all of it for the patient and family, and it's as though, if it weren't for nursing, I'm not sure families or patients would understand what's happening to them.

At all.

Right. And I don't see nurses—I think nurses may not see that as their role so much in ICU, but that to me is the heart of what we're about.

You see that as the difference the nurses make.

Oh, absolutely. You know, patients talk about, "Oh, thank you, doctor, thank you, doctor, for saving my life," but it's funny because when a patient gets taken care of in ICU, I think that more times they're seeing the ICU nurse saved my life because the ICU nurse knew when to call the doctor —

Call the doctor.

—the doctor to get something done, or you know that we are the first line of defense and their lives depend on that function that we serve.

What is it that nurses do that is unique?

You mean what do patients value the most?

That too.

Patients want to be cared for. They want you to care for them, I believe.

What does that mean?

You can give me my pills and you can give me my shots and make sure my IVs run but you better care about me. You better understand what this illness means to me and you better respond to me in a way that treats me like a human being. The nursing experience can undo a hospitalization for a patient. You know—it's like the nursing makes or breaks it for them. I believe that what patients expect from nurses is to be understood and cared about and of course it's an expectation that we would deliver the care. Ah, but I think we're expected to deliver the care "with care."

Edith Hardeman describes her perception of the role of the critical care nurse in providing competent clinical care:

There is no reason for a patient to be put in the hospital, except to receive nursing care. You can do practically everything on an out-patient basis except open heart surgery. You can go to a physician's office twice a day for ten minutes and get doctor care. The nurses are the ones that make the difference. We are there. We are eyes and ears and technology. Everything that they need, we try to be. Nurses try to be everything that the patient needs. I think that is what they are there for, observations, for interventions. Any critical care nurse who has ever worked anywhere for any length of time knows that she can manipulate whatever to get what she wants. When you get a physician to give you an order that you want, somehow it is how you asked the question. You can ask it one way and they will say no, but if you ask it another way they will say yes. I think we all have played that game, some times more than others. Sometimes not well, not to the good of the patient. We know how to work the system for the good of the patients. I think nurses are there, and nobody else is there all the time, and nurses are always there. If you need them they will stay.

What do nurses do that is most important to patients?

I think that the observation of subtle changes is probably the most important thing. I think nurses are advocates. They are the ones that are in there fighting with the lab, fighting with X-ray, fighting with the physicians, fighting with the answering services, fighting with everybody for their patients. I think that we really are there as their advocates. We listen to them, we listen to their families and to all that is going on, and we are the ones that pull it together. You are the one that takes all the little bits of information and puts it together. Is the patient telling you he is going to die this time? You are the one who synthesizes all of this and puts it all together and pictures this person as a whole. I think nurses are in the best position to see a person as a whole, realistically.

Is that unique to nursing?

I don't think that it would have to be unique to nursing. I have wrestled with that question for a long time. I don't know that any one piece could stand out as something that we do that is unique. I think that a lot of our functions are co-dependent functions. I think the thing that we do that is unique, especially critical care nurses, is that we spend the time that we do with our patients. I think our observations have to be better than those of other people, simply because we are there. I sat in a unit today and watched a man breathe for four hours, I watched his heart rhythm change, and I went downstairs and got the cardiologist and said that we need an order for two milligrams of morphine every thirty minutes for this guy. He is in bad congestive heart failure, and he is really anxious and having all this ectopy [arrhythmias], coughing and sputtering and turning purple, and he said fine. I watched him from ten in the morning until two in the afternoon. I watched that man breathe. We did not sedate him too much. We didn't put him in respiratory distress with the morphine. We gave him enough to cut down on his distress and help out his cardiac output a little bit, to give time for the Lasix [diuretic] and Aminophylline [bronchodilators] and everything else that we gave him along the way to work. We didn't want to go too far with it. I sat in a chair where I could see him and see his rhythm, and when his heart rate slowed and his breathing slowed and his color came back, then we said, 'Haven't we done well today? We have made him comfortable. We have done something good by helping this man this way." It's because we are willing to do that. We have the time and experience. We have the knowledge to make subtle observations. Every time he wakes up he is very apprehensive, his rhythm changes, his breathing gets worse, he dumps out catecholamines [adrenaline] all over the place, lots of ventricular ectopy. So when he started waking up after his acute episodes, that's when we gave him just a little bit more [morphine], and he would calm down. He did not go back into pulmonary edema. His Lasix kept working, and when he left he was looking pretty good, tuned up. I think that is what we do, we titrate things, whether it's activity or medicine or listening. I think we titrate things that they need. We try to cut down the number of visitors if they need that. We have no visiting rules in our unit. Anybody can come in and stay as long as they want. But I guarantee you, if the patient doesn't need visitors, they get thrown out, even though there are no rules. We try to gauge what they need. There is a lot of pressure because we have put it on ourselves. It is a lot of pressure to assume that you are taking care of another person's entire needs. I don't think that we do that, but we get close sometimes.

Alice Walker, thirty-one, is a pediatric critical care nurse with ten years of experience in teaching hospitals in Florida, North Carolina, and Georgia, beginning in 1978. She currently works in a children's hospital in

Atlanta and is studying for a master's degree. She describes the critical care nurse's role in the pediatric setting:

Tell me about your patients. What needs do they have?

All needs. I mean even the ones who are heavily sedated and on Pavulon [paralyzing agent] or in a coma still have emotional and spiritual needs, but yet the focus tends to be all physical in an intensive care environment. So if the physical needs are met then you've got time for the other, and it's rarely that those priorities are flipped except in the chronic child. And that's where the two focuses come. In the acute phase, especially a postoperative phase, the physical is always on the top priority, and once you get that handled, then you can talk to the child and medicate them. But they can't even have pain medication if their blood pressure is too low because it will bottom them on out until they arrest. Whereas, you might have the clinical specialist coming in standing by your bed, saying, "This child needs pain medicine." But you know in your own heart, you know you can't do that because if you give them the morphine they're just going to go right on out the door. But you know, that's because her focus is all emotional and the child—and you're the critical care nurse and yours is exactly the opposite during that time period. And that's why, if that's all you can handle and you don't have much to give emotionally or spiritually or anything to the children—that's why those nurses hate taking care of the chronic kids, because that's what you do for them. Because you're trying to normalize their environment and decrease the stimuli and not do vital signs every few minutes, and you want to just leave them there for awhile. And that's very hard for the "busy bee" critical care nurse to get used to, if you can do a whole week of one thing and then switch. But in our particular unit, they change assignments sometimes every shift that you come in. If you work three consecutive shifts you'll go from having a surgical case to a chronic kid to a dying kid in three days just like that.

And you say that's preferable in some cases.

I don't think it's preferable. I think it's awful to have to change gears that much. You can change gears like that if you're doing all acute. You can move real fast or slow down a little bit. But trying to do acute care, then going in and doing chronic care, and then doing dying care on a kid that they've practically just withdrawn all support from, all at once, is very, very hard to do.

What differences do nurses make in an ICU setting? Do you make independent decisions?

Yes and no. In the unit where I've been working more, no, because the PAs [physician's assistants] are there so much of the time. In this particular unit the PAs make all the major decisions and write the parameters. The nurses have some independent decision making, especially on influencing their decisions, but not nearly the amount that I had in my previous job, where the house officers [resident doctors] knew absolutely nothing; they rotated through once a month. So the nurses pretty much ran everything and told the house officers what to do. In this particular setting the PAs are very specialized and have been there for years and years so they're the—they do much more of the decision making than in a lot of units where there are no PAs.

So what is it that nurses do that's most important to patients?

I think experienced nurses who are used to taking care of one-service patient population anticipate things before they even happen. Even if they're not independently making decisions they are the ones notifying the people of what kinds of trends are happening, and I think the nurses pick up trends and subtle changes because they are right there all the time.

Can you give me an example?

Many times like an impending arrest where the child just doesn't look good or they're not responding the way they were. If they were a conscious child and they suddenly became very lethargic, you can pick up an impending arrest just by a feeling that you get. You know the blood pressure is still fine. You know all the vital signs look normal. The labs are all fine, but there's just something that's not quite right and many times we've called—I have—I've called the PA to come to look at this child, because there's just—his color is not good, but everything else looks fine. And sure enough by the time fifteen minutes went by they ended up having a full-blown arrest, with no explanation. The blood pressure did suddenly just fall, but at the time I called him to come see the child they thought I was nuts because everything was fine. So I think nurses who—they just—have almost like a sixth sense. It's an assessment skill I guess that's just something that they just pick up on.

What is it that nurses do, if anything, that's unique?

I think there are people that do little pieces of nursing care—and what makes the nurses unique is that they do all of that at the same time usually. They are usually doing five or six things at once instead of doing one thing at a time. Whereas a patient who is requiring respiratory therapy or physical therapy—they do that one little aspect of their care, and even if you've got respiratory therapy coming in and doing your aerosol treatments, who's the person deciding when the treatment is needed or—the nurse still does all that. They coordinate all the care that's given even if you've got a lot of ancillary help coming in; so I think, to me, the uniqueness of what nurses do, especially in critical areas is that picture that you see in some magazines where they've got eight arms, ten feet, and several different eyes coming out of the back of their heads. That to me is what characterizes them as being, not a jack of all trades *and master of none, but they really do a lot all at once, simultaneously, almost like sensory overload.*

Finally, two mature nurses speak about their perception of the nurse's role with dying patients. Each has over twenty years of experience in nursing. Their reflections mirror many of the values and attitudes evident in the reflections by younger nurses, but their experience and maturity lend a quality of comfort and empathy to their stories of patient care. Such reflections are rare in nurses over forty. Most direct patient care is provided by nurses in their twenties and thirties. Most nurses either leave nursing after a few years or pursue career paths in nursing that take them away from the bedside. Perhaps such changes as the introduction of clinical levels programs in hospitals where status and financial reward are attached to career advancement, and generally better salaries for staff nurses as a consequence of the nursing shortage, may lead to older and more experienced nurses remaining in bedside care.

Frances Larkin, forty-four, has been a nurse for twenty-two years, beginning in 1965. Currently a head nurse, she has had critical care experiences in neurology and neurosurgery, emergency room, and intensive care. She shares her beliefs about nursing care, especially about care of critically ill and dying patients.

What do you think it is that nurses do that's most important to patients?

A combination of doing what they need to have done physically and conveying the caring while you're doing it.

What about the family members?

Interpretation and the same kind of caring. And also being aware of what the patient may be going through. A lot of my time I have spent in every setting that we've just been talking about, ICU or floor or whatever, talking about the grieving process and some of the things that we take pretty much for granted, but that families don't really have an understanding of, and interpreting patient behaviors even to the patient himself, or to the family, against the background of more knowledge of what they are going through and letting them in on the "okayness" of what they're feeling.

What is it that nurses do, if anything, that's unique?

In rehab it's easy for people to perceive the nurses as the bowel, bladder, and skin person because no one else takes care of those areas. And yet what we do is —we're able to facilitate everybody being involved and having some level of understanding of that to help a patient deal with different disciplines or the systems. For instance, just the resident knowledge that you have working in a teaching hospital where it may be commonplace to us to have different levels of residents and fellows and attending physicians, but that is just so strange to a patient from a rural area who's used to seeing his country doctor every day down in Podunk hospital somewhere. And they can't sort it out and I mean they don't—it gets them crazy. But once they can understand it, or understand at least who they need to relate to, you can help a lot. It's almost like we're a person who knows enough about the different specialties and the different things that go on to help a person get—maintain—get some sense of equilibrium in the middle of it all and get them through to the other side where they can be a well person and forget that they ever were here again.

What about the use of touch by nurses?

I think that's real important. I think whether you're touching psychologically or physically, and certainly spiritually, too, is real important, because they are so isolated by the experience.

Do you have a special definition of nursing for yourself?

Well, I like the one that talks about nursing, that we deal with the person's response to his illness and I guess this is just probably my own life definition almost. In a way nursing helps make everything work, somehow work together for facilitating that patient through to the other side whether it's death or health.

Tell me about your experience with dying patients. Is that some special place that nurses can be in your experience?

Yeah. Dying patients—I'm very comfortable with dying patients because I see death as a natural process—and one that people don't get to practice up on. You know, you go through it once. I think it helps to have experienced the death of someone close to you to realize that the grief process doesn't go on for three pages in the med surg book, but maybe for three years of your life and that you never probably get to the point of what everybody calls acceptance, but more adaptation maybe, as a blind fellow told me about what he feels about the grieving process. And that you kind of just help—you kind of come alongside people and help them be there in that process and try to be what the person that's dying needs, if they happen to be family or if they're the patient—helping people realize that part of what's hard about dying, I think, is the aloneness of it; nobody else is going through it and yet if you can not be alone and can feel loved and cared about in the middle of that process that it can be a different experience.

How have you seen that facilitated or how have you facilitated that yourself?

Just with your presence and with things that you may say sensitively, not saying a lot. Sometimes standing there and being with people and crying, too, 'cause you feel their pain and not being afraid to let that part of you show.

How do you help new nurses move into those kinds of roles comfortably?

Probably a lot by role-modeling; some by talking 'cause you can kind of put some things in perspective with them. For instance, in the neuro ICU—I would generally have discussions with my newer nurses, or from time to time with my staff, about the fact that you make a choice about life, I think, and you can choose about quality and you can make a choice about quantity, and if it's just a long life, then as medical people we work as hard as we can to help that person survive at any cost; but if we're really talking about quality of whatever days any of us have on earth, then what you and I share today is it, because I may walk out of here and be dead within 24 hours. So you make a choice that with these people, even if the doctor says they've got about a week to live, I think you as a professional person have to make a choice that whatever time that person has, you are part of the quality of that and not necessarily, you know, just pushing for the quality of how long you can get them to live.

A pain-free afternoon is a realistic goal?

Exactly. 'Cause it may be their last, or it may not be. But it's kind of a choice that you have to make, I think, to be willing to go for quality versus quantity.

Back to the patients. I guess—the patient population that really gets me is neuro-related again, the head injury population, because there is so much development that a person needs when they've had a head injury in terms of just really going through developmental stages again. They are in maybe an adult body but are having to learn how to think and, hopefully, more and more, how to remember, how to eat, how to walk, how to do anything, and it's such a grief process for the patient's parents or wife or whoever it is—family. Because they are constantly reminded. It's almost like they see who they know and love and then there's this other person who comes out of that body who is very different. And it just has devastating effects on people, and it's not anything that just overnight somebody wakes up and it was like Bobby Ewing on "Dallas"—all a bad dream. It's something that goes on for years and years and causes a lot of family upheavals. Hard times.

And that patient will never be the same.

Probably won't. And people can't—I don't know how you deal with that. I just—people come to terms with that very slowly.

That's one of the hard things. I see that same kind of dynamic operating with people in crisis situations in intensive care and

**having to make decisions about initiating (or withdrawing) treat-
ment. How do you help people understand the real consequences
of treatment—spending the rest of your life on a ventilator?**

That was one thing that emergency room really helped me with. In terms
of my value system I knew this, but in terms of my experience, I came to realize
that I was not the ultimate controlling force in all of this that goes on. And
sometimes you could knock on somebody's chest three times and get 'em right
going and the other time you could work for an hour and a half and not get
'em going. To be able to be okay with my fallibility and humanity when I'm
around very heavy things has made me be free to kind of take life—and
encourage people to take life as it comes and not always have to succeed. One
of my favorite memories of the neuro ICU was a woman that we had who
wasn't a neuro patient, she happened to have an abdominal aortic aneurysm
that was enlarging—no, it was a chest aortic aneurysm. It was enlarging and
she kept breathing. She literally just had to grasp for breath, but she did this for
weeks. And I got—about the last half-year that I was in ICU we really had it
pretty much together and everything was pretty organized and I really just
went around and spent a lot of time kind of playing with the patients and
families. I mean being involved—when I say playing I mean being involved
with them at what felt like more significant levels than physical care. Sometimes
the psychosocial or spiritual dimensions, whatever. Wherever the person was
at and taking them there. And I think probably I would have loved to have
been a psychologist or social worker or whatever, but I had the little seeds of
nursing planted in me way back when. But anyway, this woman, as I began to
talk with her daughters, we kind of worked with helping her realize—helping
them realize that the twelve kids really needed to let Mama be okay with
leaving; that she was holding out so she could go home and be with them.
And they had this big family conference. All twelve of them got together by
phone or somehow, and the two daughters were designated spokesmen, and
they went into the ICU and sat on either side of her and held her hand and
said, "Mama, we know that you're really—that you said you wanted to go
home and you've been really trying to keep going so that we could let you go
home, but we need to tell you that the doctor has said that your aneurysm is
getting larger and there is no way they can surgically intervene and we need
you to know that it's okay, Mama, you don't have to fight anymore. It's okay
with us." And she just laid back on her pillow and got this serene smile on her
face, and it was within a couple of hours that she lapsed into a coma, and all
the twelve kids came from everywhere and we just got them all seated around
her and, I don't remember, I think it was maybe forty-eight hours—we would

go in and spend time—and they would talk about different things and we would go in and listen and talk and just kind of love them around her and turn her a little bit for comfort, and it was just a beautiful thing to let her make the decision to turn it loose and be okay with that and the family to do that and be involved in that. And we've had other situations, I guess with neuro and some of the brain dead patients that you see. We had situations like that that were very sweet. I don't remember how I got into talking about that. Oh yes, I was just thinking back. You said to—if patients came to mind—

Yes. What differences can nurses make with patients in those kinds of hard situations?

I think the difference in whether they hope or not. There was a lady who had been back and forth between the floor and the ICU a couple of times and was going to just about go back to the ICU again and her family had alternately gotten hopeful and then resigned and hopeful and resigned to the fact that she was going to die. I talked to her and this was many times in my head nurse role. I develop rapport fairly quickly and then am able to pretty much go to the heart of the matter with people in a very natural way that can get at some of the heavier things, it seems, without being discomforting to them. Anyway she really said what she wanted to do was go home, and she didn't want to go back to the ICU and really didn't want to stay anymore on the floor. She wanted to go home. Because she said she wanted to see her dog and she wanted to feel the wind on her face. So I talked with the daughter, who then talked with the family, who then all decided that they were going to do that, and eventually we worked it out that they took her home in an ambulance and she never reached home. But I think she left with the hope of that and it was as good as, or almost as good as, I guess getting there. And I think that the difference nurses can make is really because we're closer more often to people because of the physical care that we give or the ways that we're able to enter into their space in other ways—to really get at what's really going on with the patient. And then to be facilitators to help get that out in the open where it can be dealt with by families or doctors or whoever needs to deal with it, so that they are not so alone because they don't—someone is there and helping and caring with whatever it is they have to face.

Emily Vereen speaks of her experiences with dying patients:

What about nurturing? Is that unique to nursing?

Not really. It depends on how and who you abdicate to. You take a machine and do things. With the exception of ICUs, basic nursing care is where it starts. You could take a computer that could coordinate and plan everything that you needed to do for a patient and monitor the numbers. The difference is in that spiritual, that hands-on, that caring, that intuitive assessment that makes the critical difference in the patient. In order to do it you can't just bop in and say, "How are you?" You have got to feel, you have got to think physiologically, you have got to feel a part of that patient. You can treat a patient. I can treat your headache, but if I don't take the time to see that you have a vise around your head, then you will continue to have that headache. So nursing can make the difference in life or death for a patient from a spiritual sense. You can turn a patient around and make him want to live versus making him want to die. You can identify critical problems with that person if you want to or you can also continue to miss it if you are totally insensitive to them. If you can walk into a patient's room and he is crying you can make an assumption or you can take the time to find out why. You can say he is a pain in the butt or you can take the time to find out why.

How do you help?

What I did [with Mrs. A, see interview in the Introduction] I said, "Well I don't know, we both may be dead tomorrow. That is one question that man has not been able to answer, but I can tell you this. Nobody knows when you are going to die, that is something that we don't have. Let's talk about it. What are the things that frighten you most about dying? Is it pain? Is it being by yourself? Is it strangling? Is it throwing up? Is it nobody knowing that you died? Tell me exactly what frightens you so about dying. As human beings we know that we are going to die. Tell me if you can, what it is about death? What is frightening you right now? Not tomorrow or what you thought about yesterday. What is your fear right now?" She said, "To go by myself." I said, "Is that why you put your light on and ask for things that you really don't need? Is it that you are afraid?" She said, "Yes." I said, "Would it be reasonable for you to have a sitter, someone to come and sit with you?" She said, "Yes." As simple a task as that was—to identify that her greatest fear about dying was that she did not want to be alone. "Would you like for me to call your goddaughter, would you like for her to come?" She said, "I would." We called her goddaughter, got her up, got her lipstick on, and she said, "At least I will be pretty if I die." I told her that she wasn't going to die because we had something else to do next week. You and I have got to talk, regardless. If she goes, fine, but she is less afraid. Because so often people have fears in hospitals that are not necessary, because we don't stop to identify them. That is the nurse's role, that sensitivity. Nobody else ever asked her what was wrong. Too many human beings come across like she was. She was throwing things, ringing the bell every fifteen minutes for things like water. "Well, you have got water." "Well, I need more ice." That is a clue that something is wrong.

Did she die?

She is a tough old bird. She is going to be around. I hope I am there when she does. I really would like to be there just to be sure that somebody is there and is present because it would kill me if she were alone.

So nursing care to the patient is more the presence than doing?

It is a blend, a real blend. There is so much physiology also. We are talking skin care. We are talking positioning. We are talking body alignment. We are talking people who frequently can't move so therefore you need to have a unique understanding of stress zones and which portions of the body can be damaged. When pulling people up who have fractures, do you pull them or do you pull with a draw sheet? Basic simple things—physiology, assessment becomes very important. Patients who are using the bed pan. You need to be acutely aware of how much volume they have had in and out. Whether it is time for the Foley [catheter to drain urine], whether they need fluid or they are getting overloaded. It is an acute blend, and I think that it is not very much different except for tools than ICU nursing because it is so important to keep that patient in optimum balance regardless of whether you are going to be aggressive at life support, the person is still living. So comfort is an immensely important issue, and sometimes it requires more skill to assess without anything technological, to be able to know when Lasix [diuretic] is needed and insist to the doctor that we do need to give it because the person is ready to get to the point of drowning—and to have an acute memory about details of a person, because they aren't all written down. It is important to know and be totally observant of everything; there is nothing to help you with numbers. The nurse just has to balance and blend everything.

The nurse-patient interaction in critical care settings was described in very powerful and passionate ways by critical care nurses. The nurse was described as a humanizing link for the patient and family that assisted them in managing a return to wellness or health, recovery, or death. Nurses believed that patients who were in crisis were especially vulnerable and in need of nursing intervention. The nurse made a difference to patients through competence, caring, and management of the total care situation. The concepts of advocacy and commitment were persistent as nurses described their interactions with patients and their families.

Nurses expressed a sense of commitment to the well-being of patients. This was described as a vocation by many and was seen as quite satisfying. The value of making a difference in the lives of others was described as a privilege. Nurses were willing to use heart and mind to be what was needed for others at a given time, even at the cost of caring for themselves. This commitment was described as less a self-sacrifice than a finely developed set of skills that nurses were willing and able to use for the good of patients at a given time. Nurses, for example, performed many complex skills at one time in order to accomplish what a patient needed at a certain time — a pain-free afternoon, a peaceful death, specific medical intervention.

Advocacy was described as a complex set of roles that nurses used to act for or in place of patients or their families. The nurse in a critical care setting was the first line of defense for a sick patient. Nurses were advocates through assessment of psychological and physiological parameters and intervention to get medical help. Advocacy also implied coordination, synthesis, and integration of the patient situation. Nurses were described as the fabric of the care that holds the patient together. Nurses are there twenty-four hours a day. Nurses protect patients from consequences of illness, from poor care by others, and from hospital mismanagement. Nurses also provide emotional support to patients and families. They make the hospital system work for patients. They see subtle changes before they are trends and seek out appropriate help. They also help mobilize the patient toward wellness by decreasing fear. Finally, advocacy involves inter-preting the hospital system for patients and families.

Nurses especially valued the human link that they felt with dying patients or patients in intractable pain. Nurses often used creative methods or personal commitment to give hope and to be what a dying patient needed.

The stresses of trying to be so available to patients who might be chronically ill, acutely ill, or dying were described by many nurses. One nurse said, "There is a lot of pressure to assume that you are taking care of all of a person's needs." The satisfactions of the intimacy of nursing care seem to be achieved at a cost. The costs to nurses of this intense involve-ment with patients include the stresses of the hospital environment, the complex technology, and the potential for ethical conflict.

Technology as a stressor to critical care nurses was described in Chap-ter 2. It is but one of the perceived stressors. Others include the nature of the work itself, the hours, the demands, the perceived low self-esteem, and inadequate staffing patterns. Nurses perceived stress when factors inter-vened to prohibit them from making a difference in the lives of patients by providing the nursing care that the nurse believed was essential at the time. Nurses described a willingness to be a buffer between the patient and his or her crisis and pain and the rest of the environment. The nurse made the hospital system work for the patient, coordinated the various services for patient care, and balanced complex physiological parameters in order to stabilize a patient's status. The patient might be unconscious and dependent or awake and alert. In either case, the patient might be very sick and unstable and dependent on the nurse for critical decision making with regard to normal progress, detection, and treatment of complications, maintenance of complex drug administration, and acquisition of medical intervention if needed. Most of the time, the physician is only present at a patient's bedside if he or she has been called by the nurse. These behaviors were described as satisfying, but often also, as stressful.

The following series of interviews describe aspects of nursing practice that nurses perceived as stressful. Ways that nurses devised to manage the stress are also presented.

Beverly Quinn, 27 years old and in practice since 1982, describes the satisfactions and frustrations of critical care nursing:

What is satisfying about ICU practice?

The feeling of accomplishment, the feeling when those patients get better. That is the best part, when the patients get better and you see the improvement and/or you see the patient move to the progressive care unit. That is the most satisfying part—to see where you started out from, and how sick these patients were and what was going on with them, and to see them leave and go to the progressive care unit or to the floor.

What is the most frustrating thing?

One of the most frustrating parts is when you are short-staffed and you might have two patients and you may have to give one patient the basics and almost put them on automatic pilot. It is frustrating that these patients are so sick and you can't give them all the attention and care that you want. You can only do what is on the care plan. You need to do a cardiac output or you need to take their vital signs. You can't provide anything else for them like the psychological care or that type of thing. That is frustrating.

Why do you think nurses leave nursing?

In nursing, in general, I think one reason is that there is so much more open to women. I think that there is so much more open now. Some of the stress that nurses have to deal with, they must not have to deal with as much in some of the other professions. They say the money. They say that nurses only make $7,000 more from where they started then to where they quit. I don't think that nurses think that they have autonomy and I think that is really a stressor in the nursing profession.

Terry James, forty-one, a head nurse in an ICU, who has twenty years of nursing experience, beginning in 1967, describes the stresses of ICU practice, especially when an imbalance drives the nurse away from nursing:

What's satisfying about ICU?

I think everything about it is satisfying. I think when you look at the factors that people identify, including myself, as this is what I like about ICU—I think that when you look at the factors, this is what I hate about ICU, these are the stress points. Ultimately those get to be the same list of factors. I think that when you can really balance those, you are not too "Pollyanna" because you think everything is wonderful and you are not down in the pits because of all the stress and so forth, but you have a balance to all those. That is where the satisfaction comes from in working in a unit.

What are the stresses?

The stresses are that the patient is often unstable, the different diagnoses that your patients come in with, the knowledge of the longevity in their health problems that they are going to have when they get over this crisis point. I think the physical care is stressful, taking care of the patients, even the physical stress of doing that as a nurse. Taking care of the families is stressful. Taking care of the doctors' orders is stressful. Trying to do all the physical, the emotional care of the patient, coordinating all the other health team members to try to make sure that the patient gets what he needs, yet not bombard the patient. I think it's stressful in terms of all the knowledge that you need to work in a unit, all the technical things that you have to deal with.

Do you think that stress is why a lot of nurses leave, or do you think ICU nurses thrive on it?

I think a lot of ICU nurses thrive on that and that's why they like it and those nurses who thrive on it are also able to balance out the good and the bad. I think those nurses who leave the units have tipped the balance and the stresses are too overwhelming or they may find that just because the stresses have gotten overwhelming, that the physical and psychological damage being done to themselves is not worth that.

Celia Ingram, 39, gained a broad base of critical care experiences all over the United States, beginning in 1970—in Seattle, Chicago, Detroit, and Atlanta—as she traveled with her husband while he was in the Air Force. She describes the stresses of hospital working conditions, the relative lack of institutional support for nursing, and the stresses involved in complex patient situations:

What is stressful about ICU?

I haven't had the opportunity to work in other places but I will tell you why the city hospital is stressful. It is small. It is cramped. You cannot turn around without running into equipment or a wall. It is physically difficult. You have to move your bed in some cases to just put down the bed rail. I don't know if it was poor planning or they got the beds because they were cheap. The side rails flare out instead of what I have worked with previously, where they go straight down, which would make much more sense. When they flare out, you either run into the walls or the nightstand or the ventilator. So you are constantly pushing the bed or moving the nightstand or moving the ventilator. Medical staff changes every month. You don't get a chance to get to know anybody and learn their routines. The pay is poor. There is no peer support. You are working with agency nurses who are making much more than you are for doing the same thing or less, right? So if you are the person employed by the institution, then you are left holding the bag. It is your responsibility.

Is the institution generally supportive? Do you think that hospitals generally value the nurses that they have?

Most of them don't seem to.

Why do you think nurses leave nursing?

In many cases it is the lack of satisfaction due to poor salary or hours, or lack of peer support.

Why do you think that they leave ICU nursing?

In some cases the same things and add onto that the stresses.

Tell me about your patients—what needs do they have?

Our patients are probably some of the most complex patients that I have seen. They are indigent patients. They don't have any money. They don't have adequate housing. They don't have adequate nutrition. They don't have education. In many cases they don't have motivation to see any of these things. So they come in with a problem that for a middle-class person is hard enough. They come in with a heart attack, and you talk with them about going home and getting exercise. Well, they are sixty years old and they live upstairs in a second-floor flat and they have to walk up the stairs. It is hard enough for them to just get up the stairs. much less down the stairs, so they could walk down the street for exercise. They are just complicated. They have a lot of basic needs and those have to be met before the other complex needs. Some of these folks don't have their basic needs met. We see a lot of people that have drug dependency problems and they don't give a shit about anything. They have needs that they don't realize that they have because of their drugs.

What is it that nurses do that is most important to patients?

I think that it is patient advocacy whether or not they realize that. I have had patients thank me just for spending time with them, so evidently that is important to them. Giving them the opportunity to talk and trying to find out what they want from the treatment, not just what they need. What their expectations are.

How would you define nursing in the ICU?

I used to define it as a big clock. Used to, you had all of these things that you had to get done with all these time constraints and pressures. You don't know if this person is going to make it nor not and if you screw up it could be curtains. So it's very important, and I think that it is the heart of nursing, because you are in there really doing something for this person who is profoundly ill.

That is pretty terrifying having to deal with that consciousness. I am not so sure that that it is in the consciousness in some nurses. Do you think that it is at a conscious level?

I don't know. It should be. I had a patient one time that was supposed to be getting insulin every couple of hours, and the prior acucheck [blood sugar check done in ICU by the nurse] had been okay, and it was time for him to get the next dose of insulin. There had been a blood sugar sent down to the lab just before that, and I didn't have access to it because they were so slow and gave him the next dose of insulin. Well, there had been a mistake made along the way that I would have picked up if I had been able to get that blood test result. There had been a drop in the blood sugar, and he didn't need that insulin, and yet here he had gotten it. No wonder he was so sleepy.

Do you think that nurses provide care that others cannot?

Yes. We are back to advocacy again. I think that nurses see the whole picture. They are not just the dietitian, and interested in only how many calories the person is getting or how many calories they are expending. They are not just the surgeon, who is going to take the vein from the leg and attach it to the heart. We see the patient as a whole. Nurses should be concerned about their spiritual needs, their emotional needs, and how the whole medical team is working together to help this person get better.

What is it that nurses do that is unique?

I guess it is spending time with the patient and seeing the big picture and being able to tie it all together. Being there when the person has the questions.

Research literature talks about the use of touch by nurses and others. What is your experience with touch?

Most of the time it is very positive. I like to give back rubs and it seems beneficial and people relax when you give them a back rub. They seem to open up and be appreciative, and touch seems to open channels for the next meeting. I come in and take the blood pressure, pat the hand, ask them how they are doing. By touching they seem to know, "Yes, I care about you, and if you have a problem you let me know and I will try and help you deal with it." I think that it makes the next encounter easier. If you have developed a relationship I think that the teaching comes easier and the person is more apt to learn and work with you if this has happened.

Annie Kelly, who is working part time in a suburban hospital to maintain clinical skills while teaching nursing and pursuing a Ph.D., describes the stresses of the unknown:

What are the stresses in ICU?

If I think of a typical day when I go into work, it is the fear or the stress of the unknown. You don't know who you are going to be taking care of when you get to the unit. The fear of the unknown, of what will happen to the patient, and the worry of, "Will I be able to handle it?" I personally have anxiety about mixing medicines, setting up lines, being able to do psychomotor skills quickly enough. That is a concern to me. I can see that part-time nurses, PRN [pro re nata—as circumstances may require, as necessary] nurses, have a real concern about, "Will I be able to function efficiently enough to save the patient?" Somebody who works all the time probably would not have that fear. I never thought about it when I worked full time. I have a hard time every time I go in and there is new equipment or a new additive type drug set, a new IV line that you have to plug into this type of bottle, and I always have to get oriented to the new system every time I go into work. There is something new coming out every day. I think for full-time people, what I see them anxious about is whether they will have enough staff to take care of the patients. That is a legitimate concern, because usually you do not have enough staff. Lately when I work I don't have time to eat lunch and I am lucky if I have three minutes to run to the bathroom, and that is in an eight-and-a-half-hour day. That is unfortunate.

Do you think that the nature of your work itself is stressful?

No, I don't think so for critical care nurses. They have that personality type. That is why they have chosen that area because that is what they enjoy. For other nurses that are not in that area it would be very stressful to take care of patients who are that sick. But for critical care nurses, and for me too, it is a real challenge and we like challenges.

You don't see any critical care nurses in their sixties. Why is that? What are your goals?

I plan on staying involved in critical care, but not on a full-time basis. I will be honest with you. I project that within the next three to five years that critical care nursing staff in hospitals will be part time and PRN people. That there is no way, except for a few select individuals, that people can work that forty-hour week in that environment and maintain their sanity and have a family life. I think again that it would have to be part-time or PRN and nothing else because the stress is just too much.

You say the stress is too much. Why?

The stress, the decision making, trying to fit it all in, all the technical, psychological and physiologic care you have to give to the patient, and you have to document it during an eight-and-a-half-hour period.

The work is not inherently stressful, but what I hear you saying is that the job is stressful?

Getting it all done in the time, mainly because of staffing. If the critical care units were appropriately staffed, then the job would not be as stressful. I don't foresee any additional staffing than the two-to-one ratio that we have now. Many times when I go in we need a one-to-one on every patient and we have two patients to one nurse and that is just too much, but that happens consistently. Because of that I won't go into critical care full time. Pay-wise I think more nurses will be going into it part time or like this Baylor time, where they could have consistency on a Monday through Friday job and every other weekend, that would help in de-stressing yourself. If you either have the same two days off every week or you just work weekends. That definitely helps take care of the stress when you have to go and take care of two critically ill patients in one eight-hour period. Versus the old method of staffing in critical care that you would have every other weekend and you would get your other days off one day a week. That definitely does not promote getting rid of stress. You don't see old critical care nurses except for possibly head nurses, which is unfortunate because they are not working and tuned in to the needs of the younger nurses. I don't think that you will see old nurses in critical care. I have met no nurses that are in their forties and fifties and sixties because they feel they cannot keep up with the technology. I plan on continuing to work in the unit until whenever because I have fun when I go to work now, and I never did before.

Sara Ryan, thirty, a nurse since 1978, is a Black critical care Army nurse. She describes the stresses of being "everything" to a patient or family:

What was appealing to you about ICU?

I think one of the reasons that I really did like it was because a lot of people looked up to you and physicians respected your opinion and they respected your education, assessments, and what you told them about patients. Not that ward nursing is bad. I enjoyed it while I was there. I have trouble now working on a ward because I can't get myself organized for more patients. I just like intensive care better. I'm just tired of it. I don't know. It is the same stress over and over again.

What is stressful about it?

Okay, patients dying and you have to deal with the patient's family. They want you to be their loved one's savior. They look at you like, "Can't you do something?" and it is more so the nurses than the physicians that they depend on. They ask nurses questions that they would not dare ask the physician. I guess that it is because we are easier to talk to.

Can you give me an example or a specific patient?

I had one man who had fallen off of a water tower and fractured all the ribs on the right side of his body and they thought that he had a vertebral fracture. He kind of broke everything on the right side of his body. They brought him to Martin Army Hospital, which is a community hospital and we don't have that much in the way of sophisticated equipment. But we have the basics so that we can take care of somebody. The wife had questions about his mental status because he drank a lot and sometimes when he would get drunk and wake up from his hangover he would be confused and would say off-the-wall things. The lady would tell me that, even though he would do that, he now seemed different. Because I did not know him I did not know what she was talking about. He was not intubated at the time, but she would say that he was not talking right. She kept telling me this, and I would tell her to talk to the doctor the next time he came around and tell him what you are saying. I would have told him for her but I did not know the subtleties of what she was saying. That is what I mean. They look to you to answer all of these questions for them. He did have a subdural hematoma. After we found that out we had to transfer him to a neuro hospital and we had to intubate him later on because he started having respiratory problems, which they probably should have done in the first place because the man had all of his ribs fractured and he was a smoker, too. For her, I was her focal point. Maybe it was because I was Black and she was Black and maybe that is why she was always coming to me with these things. They come to you with problems that—maybe I should not say they aren't the patients' problems, but "How am I going to pay for the electricity?" and stuff and you have to go to social workers for them and tell them where to go to get this taken care of and where to go to get these benefits from. That kind of thing. They kind of become your children and you have to look after them and take care of them.

The nurse takes care of everything?

Everything, that is what is expected of them. That is what you are supposed to do. It is not like something extra that you are doing. It is something that you are expected to do. They ask you for your phone number at home so they can call you and that kind of thing.

And that is stressful?

Yes, it is stressful to know that you have somebody that dependent on you. That is what I have found. It happens a lot. I don't know if it is because of the military promoting this kind of dependency of its dependents. You know what I mean by dependents? Dependents are the people who are the family members of the active duty people, and I think that is something that the Army promotes—for dependents to be dependent on the system. I really think that is it.

You are part of the system?

An officer, and in nursing, and I am supposed to be able to solve everything or know how to solve everything.

You are a captain?

Yes, I am a captain now. I really was getting a little stressed out and burned out on nursing. I have been doing bedside nursing for quite awhile now and shift working gets tiresome, working with men gets tiresome, and you want a change. I don't care. I always hear, "I want to go to graduate school so I can be near the patients." I think that is a crock of stuff. You get tired of that all the time. You want to do something different with your life, and you want your life to be normal, whatever that is. Work nine to five and have your weekends off and spend your holidays with your family. I have not had a Christmas off since I have been in the Army.

Carla Olson describes some of the satisfaction and stresses in coping with critically ill patients in a highly technical environment, and the stress-reducing components and the rewards of making a difference in the lives of patients:

What do you think is satisfying about CCU practice today?

Well, when you are not doing heart transplantation, you feel a lot of rewards with limiting infarct size and seeing people go home in three days when it would have been two weeks, if you are old enough in nursing to know what the alternative was. And if you see infarcts you feel some satisfaction in getting people through that even though the quality of life is going to be reduced afterwards. You feel some feeling of contribution to the fact that they survived. With transplants the rewards are more when the patient gets the heart. You get that type of reward that is terrific, but at the same time that reward comes, there is this fear that the patient is going to try to remain dependent on you, to stay in contact all the time and have anniversary parties and that kind of stuff, which makes you uncomfortable in some way. But there is so much loss involved in that transplant process that the rewards become debatable and whether they are worth the in between that you have been through. Because it is difficult to feel joy for one patient when someone you worked with recently didn't get that, and it's very difficult to keep both in perspective. Why one? Why not the other? So it just depends on what you are doing.

What are the frustrations? You addressed some of them.

Well, our overall frustration is that the medical staff are practicing some of this modern-day technology, but with a hang-over of their old patterns, which kind of makes it seem schizophrenic to me. We have got a lot of transition to go through with the physicians, those who are truly entrenched in a different kind of medical care and don't want to go into transplantation in contrast with the ones who are going to be, hopefully, providing very detailed, very sophisticated, invasive kind of support, minute to minute. We want those people who are doing that to have enough moral background that they would not do it when it's not appropriate, and to be able to go through an evaluation of how far should we go with this patient and have that be realistic and not out of touch with what's reasonable for that patient's options.

Why do you think nurses leave ICU nursing or coronary care?

I think that when they're forced to take care of people for whom there is no hope, that's the worst of it. I hear and see that in some ICUs. They've got people for whom there really is no hope and yet they are still flagging away—ventilator patients, and at this point in time the culture really doesn't make it easy for you to back off, and people still expect the medical profession to cure anything. So I don't know what will happen in the next generation, but my guess is they are going to have to be more selective of who they go that far with. I think at that point, it will seem more normal for the ICU nurse, that it's either worth it or it isn't worth it and her judgment of what's practical will be the same as what the patient and family choose, too. But at this point the physicians and patients and the families aren't given an option. They just keep persevering in the face of enormous adversity with no reason to expect to get any hope, but yet they keep doing it. For example, we had a patient with AIDS on a ventilator and he was in ICU for weeks. I just don't know how you can justify that, if there is absolutely no sign in the world that they are going to get off and in a lot of situations like that that the nurse herself was very clear. You knew it was hopeless, but the physicians had gotten caught in the scenario of some form of life support and didn't know how to get out of it. I sort of respect the brain death phenomenon where the physician says that the patient is legally dead. I'm taking off the ventilator whether you like it or not, and I think somehow it will come to that in the next transition of things. It will be more accepted culturally that you don't go further than that because it isn't reasonable, it's not practical. I think that nurses have to feel like what they are doing is worthwhile and that's some of it. But yet some of it is just the fact that the system doesn't acknowledge the stress that it involves physically and emotionally and provide enough rewards to balance that, in money or whatever it would take to limit your work week, anything that would make it possible for you to continue to do it and feel good about it. The system just doesn't do that. They address 40 hours in ICU, the same as 40 hours in an outpatient cath lab, and there isn't any attempt to compensate for higher levels of tension or whatever.

What do you think the stresses are? You addressed some of them.

I think some of it revolves around torture, the things you are doing to people that you know have some painful consequences and yet you don't have any choice. I think it does something to you after a while, but you just don't want to do it again. Some of the repulsive things you have to deal with over and over.

Like what?

Oh, specimens, sputum, all the folderol with isolation techniques, and all that barrier kind of stuff with AIDS, to try to keep yourself safe, and I think people can tolerate a little bit of it, but there comes a point where it's very old, if you don't feel like you are getting something special in order to tolerate those things. I think the inevitable accountability that the families and the patients have, their expectations, their demands are foisted on the nurse somehow, and that pressure gets to be old.

You mentioned earlier that people expect the medical system to fix everything?

And you go through that with every family until they finally accept that there isn't anything else that can be done, and that gets old, having to sort of admit failure on a regular basis. I just think it's a business in the sense that institutions need to measure what they are asking people to do against what the community considers acceptable versus not acceptable behavior and then reward them accordingly, so that they know that it's understood that they are dealing with irritable, difficult people and because of that their salary is such and such, or they get a week in the Bahamas every six months, you know, something that really says clearly to the employee, I know it's a high-stress job and for that reason we are compensating you this way or providing you this relief. You know like massages at the end of the shift for any nurse taking care of a level five [very ill] patient, or just anything to attempt to give credit for what you had done. If you had taken care of a patient with this complexity of illness you get something extra, you get a day off every once in a while, or—There's just no acknowledgment now that if you pass pills and chart it on four patients on the floor, and work your 40 hours without any big deal, that that's any different than if you work that same 40 hours with a patient with cardiomyopathy who's been about to drive you to drink, you know, constantly, and you're so physically and emotionally burned out that you can't even think. There is just no address of that in the system, so the inequity gets to people, regardless of what they are actually getting paid, but the fact that there is inequity and they are not getting any direct recognition for it. So people just get tired of not having a reward and seeing that they are working five times harder and it's costing them more than someone in another spot, and sooner or later they get smart enough to realize that and remove themselves from it.

Vera Strickland agrees with Olson that feeling that the work is worthwhile and that nurses made a difference to patients is stress-reducing for nurses:

Getting involved with people in the way that we're talking about is stressful too.
Yeah, it's a different sort of stress.
Yeah, but is also rewarding, what about that?
My belief is that even though it all is stressful, I think if we can see somewhat of the impact of what we do and it does make a difference, it alleviates some of that stress. And I say that just from some experiences we had. When we first introduced the concept of primary nursing and first started that, there was a lot of fear, there is a lot of accountability in that, but it just seems like there was more accountability, a lot of hesitation. But one of the young staff members who was most resistive to change, who was most resistant to us

starting that, after we had been doing it for a period of two or three months, came to me and said, "I want to tell you, I kicked against this, but I will never work in another unit in which they are not doing primary nursing, and I will personally talk with any other unit where you want to start it. I'm absolutely sold on it." I had another staff nurse who had been working with us, sharp kid, been working with us about three years, and I saw her one day when she had dismissed a patient and she was rolling the wheelchair back up, and I just happened to come up, walk alongside with her and ask how things were going. She says, "You know that's the first time in three years I've been working on that floor, I felt like I sent a person home that I really knew and that I was able to make a difference in his life and his recovery." So just picking up on those two experiences make me believe that we like to see what we do make some impact. Not just for right now. I think that's one reason why some of the most prestigious positions in nursing tend to be those in which you have crisis intervention, I mean as I understand it, flight nurses are the most prestigious today. By your doing something, that what you do you get instant feedback on, instant gratification that you've made a difference. So whether it's the instant or whether it's the long haul, I think that's one of the things as nurses begin to feel that their own competency makes a difference.

Alice Walker introduced on p. 109, describes the stresses of critical care and how involvement in family over a period of time can reduce stress and increase the feelings of satisfaction:

What's your experience of touch in patient care, with the kids, in critical care settings?

Oh, a tremendous amount is used. Even the infants who are hooked up to every piece of equipment you can imagine, the one thing they do respond to best is rubbing their heads or just—you can pick them up and put your hands all the way under their backs, and rock them a little bit or just pick them up about six inches off the bed—even with all the equipment on—and they will calm right down if they're used to it. Now some of them get adverse to any kind of touch if they've been in there very long, but the acute kids do much, much better by being touched and talked to. Even those soft, real squishy, fuzzy animals. You can take them and curl them around their heads, or lay them right by their bodies just so they can feel something on them and they'll just lie there real still. And if they are just lying out flapping in the breeze with air blowing over them, they are just agitated all the time. Same thing with blankets. Sometimes with all the chest tubes in them you can't swaddle them.

But infants are used to being bound up almost in a fetal position where they are real secure, and when you put them on the Ohio bed warmers, which are used in most of the intensive care units, they are tied with their arms straight out and their legs straight out like little frogs and there's no security in that. So if you can figure out a way to bundle even just their legs with an IV in it that you have to be looking at all the time—they'll be much, much calmer than if they're just tied straight out. They don't fidget near as much because they feel a little bit more—bundled and secure.

What's satisfying to you about critical care?

Hmmm. I think the most satisfying thing is direct patient care even though I do a fair amount of teaching in my current job and have always done that. I think the reason that part is satisfying is because it lets the nurses that I teach be able to take better care of their patients so they're better satisfied with their own care. Because nothing is more frustrating than to have to do something you don't understand or having no rationale for doing a procedure because that's the way it's always been done. And that's the way I tend to teach. If you know why, then you'll remember why and do it that way. If I understood it, then I could do it, no matter how hard it was to do. If I had some kind of knowledge base that was a little bit better than what I'd had before with the same kind of patient I always felt like I did a better job. So I think that the satisfying thing is giving good quality care no matter what the outcome is. If you felt like you gave good quality care and nothing happened because of that—you know, even if the patient has a cardiac arrest and dies—if you were over with another patient and you weren't spending time with your own there is always a twinge of guilt there. What if I was over there doing what I was supposed to be doing, would this have happened? And nobody will ever know the answer to that, but if you were there on the spot and felt like you gave good quality care, then those feelings don't usually come because you know it was one of those things that happen because you saw it happen right before your very eyes. But if you're short-staffed and you're over there doing something, but you felt like you should have been over there with your other patient, then you're just devastated because you think it is sort of your fault that the whole thing happened.

What are the frustrations about critical care?

Inadequate staffing. The quality of care takes a huge dive any time there is inadequate staffing. The liabilities associated with that—with the decreased quality of care and the short staffing. Our intensive care unit in the last six to ten months has been 50 percent staffed by floor nurses who have never been in an intensive care unit before. One of the things that makes it less frustrating is when you have a free and floating charge nurse, which is a new concept that's developed over the last five to ten years. A long time ago one person who had her own patient assignment was designated as being in charge and was supposed to be supervising everybody in there—all the patient care and taking care of her own patient load. And that's physically impossible to do in a critical care unit. Maybe on various floors that's possible where they have a huge amount of time. But units that I've worked in that had free charge nurses that had no patient care responsibilities, where they could float and help where they were needed, really did know what was going on because they could come by and see things in your patient care and point them out to you, you know, without making you feel like a dummy, who would help you when you weren't seeing things. And that also enhanced the quality of the patient care because you had two people's eyes looking at the same problem, instead of one, where you were just the Lone Ranger by yourself. So when short-staffing problems occur—the first thing they'll do is take the charge nurse and give her a patient assignment, or when you've got that heavy load of floor people in there, float nurses that have never worked in your area, the charge nurse's time is sucked up by trying to keep those people from hurting anything.

Why do nurses leave nursing, particularly ICU nurses?

Ah . . . all the friends that I've had that have left, left because those types of frustrations, I just mentioned. They reached a point to where they felt there was a no return from that.

Ah huh.

One girl, I know in particular, now is doing a business degree not only for pursuing more money, but the money end of it to her is very frustrating. She's been in nursing for fifteen years and makes no more than . . . well, she makes more than she did when she started but not substantially more. So that's why she's doing that. And then she's just received repeated frustrations, even though she's got that much experience she's on the same level as all the other people, rotating shifts, and there are no . . . brownie points for any kind of seniority. So to her, that's frustrating to know that she's doomed to work nights forever.

You say you can concentrate on the nursing care—what is it?

The nursing care to me is divided two ways. If you've got these acute kind of patients, then it's very high level assessment and . . . very autonomous. You work within parameters they've set for you to maintain a patient's physical level. Usually the first day after open heart surgery mental status is not as much of a problem because they are very, very heavily sedated. Your main concern is pain relief and sedation because you don't want them wiggling and jumping around and causing bleeding. The children bleed much more than the adults do who have a similar kind of surgery because their bypass time and the length of the surgery is sometimes six hours, instead of a couple, like they are in and out on an adult. So those particular kinds of patients are to me very challenging and you can enjoy taking care of them, because the next day when you come back to work they're ready to have all that equipment taken off and they're fine unless something major has happened. But then there is the other set of them that don't do well, who come back upstairs with their chests still open—they leave them open for a couple of days—and they end up having kidney failure and everything else, so even if they end up recovering they're harder to take care of because it's more of a chronic, you don't see the light at the end of the tunnel kind of patient. Now some of those do recover, but a large percentage of them, if they have that many major complications within the first 24 to 48 hours, they do not do well and they end up being in the unit for a month or more. And they don't come off the ventilator. They end up with such bad pulmonary edema. When you come into that particular unit you can have one or the other kind of patient. And the nurses who like the area usually fight over who gets "the good patient" and who has to take the cruddy ones, because most of the nurses who work in that area do not like chronic care. There are a few who have gotten into primary care where they really establish a rapport with a family, but our particular kinds of patients from referrals do not have real . . . there are a few . . . but the majority of them don't have good families, they're usually not even there at all, or if they are, they're so poor or ill educated that you can't feel like you can do a lot with the family. You spend more time just repeating things over and over or sending them back to the waiting room so that it's not something that you get a lot of satisfaction out of that would make taking care of a chronic kid over and over a rewarding experience.

Ah huh.

And in fact I've only had one patient where that really paid off, where I felt really a benefit from. I took care of a patient who was in the unit 21 days, every shift that I was there, except one, I think. On days and nights, I rotated through both. And at that time . . . the family was real nice and it ended up being a mother who I went to high school with who I did not know in high school. But when we started talking about where we were from, we suddenly realized that we had gone to the same high school, but we had been on split sessions, so I had not seen her because she was in the other session. But anyway we just had some mutual contacts and knew a few similar people and ended up talking, and their baby had two surgeries during this course of the stay. They were very well educated and very interested and wanted you to explain things over and over to them because they wanted to understand every little thing. So you felt like you were making a big difference in their outlook on the whole situation, besides just taking care of the infant. And the baby was a beautiful baby and should have done well through the other surgery so it wasn't one you just give up on from day one either. So because of that and the parents made the difference because they would always ask, "Who's going to have my baby on this shift," and they would request who they wanted. So they even had an influence on which nurses got him and they liked me from day one because they had some kind of personal identification with me and one other nurse. There were two of us. So we ended up basically doing a primary care on this infant, and he ended up dying at the end of this twenty-one-day period. And it so happened that I was taking care of him the shift that he died and I had to call the parents at home to come into the hospital when he was having an arrest. But because I was their nurse and was their consistent person, they were not really as upset as if it were a different nurse. Because every time a different nurse took care of him and some major incident happened, like when he had to go back to the OR [operating room] for the other surgeries, a little twinge of them blamed that nurse, you know. Well, what did she do wrong that you wouldn't have done? And nothing really happened that way, but they were real anxious. So just a familiar face lowered their anxiety tremendously even though the whole situation was at its height. So anyway, that situation went on and that day was real hard for me because I had gotten real attached to those parents. And I didn't usually get—there were a few over the course of the ten years that I'd gotten attached to, but not quite so much as these people. And I think it was because it ended up going way back into my past and pulling out something that I had not ever experienced—. So the next day she called—and I had never gone to a child's funeral—it's something that colleagues of mine had done that I just never had any inkling to do, but she called me the next day after the funeral and asked me if it would be okay if she called me in a month or so or could she have my address and send me a note in the mail and I said, "Sure." It was real surprising—she had called to see if I was all right at the hospital. To check on me, to see if I was okay. And I thought, boy, this is really unusual for this mother to do that.

And you did go to the funeral?

I didn't. She called me the next day after the funeral. And I had never had a parent call me back to see how I was doing, you know. Because, like I said, it had been a big ordeal that whole morning when the arrest went on forever. They did make it to the hospital before he died. And the grandparents and everybody. I knew the whole entire family. And then I left the next week to go on a snow skiing trip and when I came back. Oh, while I was gone I sent them a card. I had gotten their address and just took it with me on my little vacation and sent them a card with a little note, but I'd done that in the past. But I still didn't think a whole lot about it. It was something I wanted to do, but it wasn't a huge big deal. When I came back she called me and wanted to know if we could get together for lunch one day, if it wouldn't bother me. But she said she had been in this "tizz" the whole time and just felt like she didn't understand half of what went on and she just needed to sit down and ask me some questions if I didn't mind answering them because her husband had been real supportive through the whole crisis and since the baby's death had gone berserk. And he was no help at all. So here's when she was needing support and he was no help at all. He couldn't even explain to her the things that he had been understanding during the hospitalization that had just gone over her head. So we did. So I thought what can it hurt? So it ended up that through the next year we talked periodically on the phone. And she lived real close to where my parents lived. And so when I'd go up there, occasionally we'd meet for lunch at the mall. And that went on, I guess for about nine months after the baby had died. And then they had another baby this August and made me the godmother of the new baby and called me the guardian angel. And so we developed a real close relationship, over not just the baby's death, but over the whole entire experience. Because they had waited eight years to have that first baby and just thought they would never have another one. And he was an eight-pound, normal-looking baby, except for having this real severe heart defect. That was a really neat experience that I normally don't have. When I teach new nurses I don't recommend they develop those kinds of rapport with every patient because you'll just get totally burned out if you have to deal with something that heavily emotional every time. In this particular case it helped me as much as it helped the family. And I think that's the difference. A lot of times if you the nurse gets attached to a family or patient and they're not so attached to you it's more of a one-way street. And then you end up being a bad reminder to the family because a lot of families, once they've had a child die—they don't even—Even when they come back for the autopsy conference they won't even walk up to the intensive care unit. We've had a couple of parents who will come back occasionally just to speak to one or two nurses, or they'll send cards. They usually always send cards or flowers to the staff that took care of their child. But that's about all they can handle. They won't walk through the doors of the hospital sometimes for years down the road. But if a family does indicate they need that and the nurses are willing to do it, I think if it's a two-way thing, then I think somebody else could have as positive an experience as I had. I mean, that gave me strength to take care of any number of those same kinds of kids for years after that, because of seeing that I made a difference. Even though the child had died and I thought he should have done fine—that he would have been one of the ones that we corrected that did well—and he didn't, I still did not see defeat in the whole situation because the parents ended up growing and getting something out of my care.

What was it that you did that made a difference?

Well, the things that she has told me that she remembers from the hospitalization experience was my being honest and taking the time to explain things to them over and over again if they didn't understand, and treating them as intelligent human beings who were concerned about their child rather than just telling them what I thought they needed to know. You know, answering them and telling them and teaching them things. That's what she said was the most supportive. And because I knew the family and I'd taken care of the child for two or three weeks I knew where they were at. It was almost like I could tell what to say at the right time and the right place kind of thing.

What about in the lunch meeting you had—the first one?

About all I did was go over the same things I'd gone over in the hospital that at the time she didn't remember—you know, this happened, and then this happened and—how that all was hooked together, and did that mean, you know, this—she would have questions about the sequence of events. The surgery happened first. Why did they have to do the second surgery? Why did they not notice that the baby had this defect before it was born? And having to explain how those changes happen in the delivery room, because she brought pictures from the delivery room to show me what the baby looked like without tubes and ventilators and stuff, which is the way she wanted to remember the baby, which is fine. But having to just explain some of those things. So it was just mainly reassuring and explaining things that she knew the answers to, but just was real confused on.

So why do you think that that kind of involvement contributes to burnout? Particularly in new nurses?

In new nurses, I think if it's that kind of involvement, it wouldn't contribute to burnout. But what tends to happen to new nurses is they pour their hearts and their energy into something like that without that kind of a return and so without the return at the end of that is where you just drain yourself. Because you just cannot put that amount of energy into a unit where you might take care of six kids over a six-month period who go through that same kind of experience. It's not like it's one a year. It can be very high numbers and . . .

So just the stress of dying children, or the stress of the work itself—?

And just—I just have always strongly believed that you needed to deal with it in a different way than you would your own family member. And see, if you go to the funeral and grieve with the family, that's more like you are treating them as if they're part of your family and you need to do it in two different ways, or that was the way I was trying to teach the new staff. You know—you can't go through this just as if it were your own family every time. You've got to deal with it on a little bit more professional level. Not that crying is wrong. I've never, ever believed that. I mean at the time. It's the continual attachment to the child and the rituals of society—and occasionally some of the nurses who did do those things coped fairly okay. But not usually. Any of the ones who made a definite habit of always going to all those children's funerals and keeping up with the parents and stuff had a pretty high level of stress and burnout symptoms that were just typical at the time.

How do you think nurses cope with the stress in ICU?

All different ways. They—it depends on their personalities. The nurses who are real active types who have a lot of outside interests, I think, work through their own stress well. Because they don't go home and brood over it, or take all of the ICU home with them. They can kind of leave it at work and then they are excellent nurses when they are there but they don't constantly live it.

They have a separate life.

Yeah. They have a separate life. Exactly. The nurses who did not have much of an outside social or personal life did very badly with the stress. Work was their whole life and so, when the unit was in a real down time and all the patients were doing poorly, they were in the same boat; and when everything was going well, they were fine. But they didn't have enough outside interests to have a balance. And so I think that the balance—even if it's—it doesn't have to be really socially related. Some of the ones who were active athletes and ran and jogged and were into exercise, they did okay too. It wasn't because they were social butterflies that they did well, it was just having a balance in their lives so that it wasn't all their eggs in one basket. And I—that's me too. I do the same thing.

Clearly, as the critical care unit evolved and became more specialized, complex, and highly technical, the nursing role changed in many significant ways. The nurse became the central feature and resource in the critical care unit—uniquely identifiable because of refined skills, a new aggressiveness in promoting patient advocacy, and emerging roles, which included coordinating the care of these very ill patients. Although the environment and many of the roles and skills were new, the critical care nurse incorporated them into the traditional roles and relationships that nurses have always had with patients. Thus, the tasks and responsibilities were additive. The consequences of these changes have in some cases increased the status and self-concept of nurses and nursing and in others have precipitated almost a schizophrenic ambivalence about nursing practice. Certainly the experiences shared in the interviews make visible many of the outcomes of the changes brought about by the evolving critical care environment.

As nursing shared in the positive outcomes of technology, it also shared in the lack of clarity in roles and relationships and the ethical dilemmas that increasingly occurred with highly technical interventions with patients. Nurses were a consistent presence with patients and families in these latter situations and had to forge new ways of coping with patients who did not do well.

One of the major outcomes of the critical care environment was the persistence of stress. Nurses described many aspects of critical care nursing as stressful. The work itself, often physically difficult, requires rapid, complex decision making and the outcomes have the potential of being life-threatening. Knowing the seriousness of the tasks, many nurses described a fear of the unknown. Further, great demands are routinely placed on the nurse by patients, families, physicians, and nurse administrators. The assumption of these responsibilities by nurses in these situations is often not rewarded but expected as a part of the job. The critical care environment, shift work, low salaries and limited opportunities for advancement, low staffing and the liabilities associated with it, and dealing so constantly with both dying patients and the patients who represent medical failure are other factors discussed as stressful by critical care nurses.

One of the most frustrating and stressful situations described by many of the nurses who were interviewed involved the feelings associated with inflicting torture or ongoing painful treatments on patients for whom there was no hope of return to any quality of life. Similarly, seeing patients do well, or survive or increase their quality of life, was described as very rewarding and satisfying. Nurses often established meaningful reciprocal relationships with dying patients and their family members that generated personal satisfaction and a renewed energy to cope with further stressful patient situations. Even if patients died, or deteriorated, nurses felt satisfaction if they saw the impact of their own competency. Nurses felt rewarded if they made a difference and felt that what they had done with patients was worthwhile, even if the activities associated with nursing care were stressful.

Nurses reduced stress by finding ways of "making a difference" with

4. The Ethical Dimensions of Critical Care Nursing

The ethical issues described by critical care nurses reflect all the dimensions of critical care settings described in earlier chapters. The setting, the rapidly changing technologies, and the evolving roles of nurses in critical care settings, all influence the ethical dilemmas that confront nurses, patients and their families, physicians, administrators, and many others who have prolonged contact in hospital settings.

Society is more and more bombarded with the consequences of contemporary medical treatment. The syndrome of multiple system failure and death from gradual deterioration and/or catastrophic events in a highly technological ICU (intensive care unit) setting is increasingly common. The social, financial, and human costs are immeasurable in such varied aspects of health care as organ procurement for transplants, fetal organ and tissue donation, and experimentation; treatment and privacy rights of patients with acquired immune deficiency syndrome (AIDS) and drug resistant tuberculosis (TB) versus risk to the public health, including the well-being of health care workers; reproductive issues such as contraception, abortion, surrogate parenting, extrauterine conception, and artificial insemination; and the rights of the aged in our society to health care. Issues of quality of life, death with dignity, right to die, and euthanasia emerge with increasing frequency in the treatment and care of terminally ill, dying, comatose, and brain dead individuals. Rapid changes in technology often seem to outpace the redesigning of social and legal structures and moral thought.

All these issues are influenced by problems and inequalities in U.S. society with regard to resource allocation and access to medical treatment. The economics of health care are tied to political and legislative processes and health policy. At the present time, many groups in the United States are underserved because of reduced or terminated services, especially the urban poor, women, particularly pregnant women, children, and minorities. This has consequences for institutional acute care. For example, a decrease in federal or state funding for antepartal care reduces the number of out-patient services in urban areas. As a consequence, pregnant teenagers often receive no prenatal care. These women are already at high risk because of their age and frequently because of drug use or poor nutrition. Increasing numbers of these teenage mothers receive their first medical attention when they arrive in labor in an emergency room. In addition, many hospitals may turn a woman away if she has no proof of insurance. The risk is damage to mother and baby entailing a much higher financial burden to the individual, hospital, and society in terms of prematurity, neonatal ICU care, and long-term care of mentally or physically challenged children and adults than would be the cost of preventive prenatal care of the mother. Similarly, out-patient care for a child with asthma is much cheaper than emergency room care, hospitalization, or intensive care treatment of a child with respiratory distress. The consequences of these health care policies have changed the population of patients seen in hospital settings in the 1990s. Patients are older, younger, sicker, and in more distress prior to seeking treatment than in previous years.

Howard E. Freeman et al. (1987: 6–18) report the results of a 1986 study conducted by the Robert Wood Johnson Foundation about access to and use of health services in the United States between 1982 and 1986. The study reported that the gap in medical care between urban and rural residents had diminished and that most Americans were satisfied with their physician and in-patient hospital care. Overall use of medical care by Americans had declined in terms of hospitalization and physician visits. Access to physician care for individuals who were poor, Black, or uninsured had decreased, particularly for those in poor health. Hospitalization had also decreased for disadvantaged groups, but at a rate comparable to that of the general population. However, the uninsured and Black and Hispanic Americans received less hospital care than might be appropriate, given their higher rates of illness. Underuse of dental and medical services by key groups was reported; these groups included pregnant women in the first trimester, patients with diagnosed hypertension, and persons experiencing symptoms of significance such as bleeding (other than nosebleeds, menstrual periods, or bleeding caused by accident), shortness of breath after light exercise, loss of consciousness, chest pain, and unexplained weight loss of more than ten pounds. These findings confirm the growing problems of access of underserved groups to health care in the United States.

Critical care nurses are directly involved with the sickest patients in the

American hospital system. They are also at the forefront of the ethical issues that have emerged as a consequence of treatment in critical care settings. These situations are complex, and the issues often are not clear. Simple logic and right or wrong judgment are insufficient as models of problem solving or analysis.

This chapter portrays the range of ethical dilemmas that critical care nurses have articulated as significant in their practice. The ethical dilemmas described by these nurses cover the following broad areas: issues related to death with dignity for dying patients, especially in circumstances associated with "do not resuscitate" (DNR) orders, realities surrounding organ transplant, and problems of resource allocation. Background material on ethical decision making will precede the presentation of the interview data and discussion.

Ethics is defined as the body of moral principles or values governing good, evil, duty, and obligation in a particular culture or group (*Webster,* 1988: 426–427). For example, in the United States infants are generally protected by social and legal codes, whereas in some cultures, infanticide is an acceptable method of population control. Morality in a given culture reflects the complex relationship between needs and rights. Many factors influence whether need fulfillment is a right, how persons are treated in a given society, and how the legal structure becomes formalized to reflect the social values. For the purposes of this discussion, ethics is understood in the Socratic tradition. Ethics is an attempt to formulate systematic responses to the question: What, all things considered, ought to be done in a given situation (Benjamin and Curtis, 1992: 9)? Ethical inquiry in health care presumes a cognitive process of analytical decision making; a knowledge of legal, religious, and cultural constraints; and a consideration of role relationships, institutional constraints, and dependent, independent, and co-dependent functions of physicians and nurses.

Several writers in recent years have provided new insights into ethical issues in nursing practice. Anna Omery (1989: 499–508) clarifies and defines values, moral reasoning, and ethics in nursing practice. Ketefian (1989: 508–522) reviews and critiques measures and tools of moral reasoning and ethical practice in existing nursing research and concludes with very useful suggestions for future research. Elizabeth C. Reisman (1988: 789–802) and Christine Grady (1989: 523–534) address ethical principles related to nursing care of HIV-infected persons. These issues include, but are not limited to, the moral obligation to provide care and confidentiality (Reisman) and courage to face risks and impartiality to temper prejudice (Grady).

A five-step model of analysis for ethical decision making is presented by Martin Benjamin and Joy Curtis (1992: 12–19). First, they suggest, determine and obtain relevant factual information. Second, aim for clarity and draw relevant distinctions. Third, construct and evaluate arguments. Fourth, develop a systematic framework. Fifth, anticipate and respond to objections.

Increasingly, ethics committees exist in hospital settings to assist physicians, administrators, nurses, patients, and families with resolution of very complex ethical issues. In 1972, the American Hospital Association published "A Patient's Bill of Rights," delineating twelve areas of patient rights and hospital obligations, including the right to considerate, respectful, and continuous care; the right to information about diagnosis; the right to informed consent; the right to refuse treatment; the right to privacy; the right to reasonable treatment; and the right of access to the hospital record (Benjamin and Curtis, 1992: 182–183). Articulation of these rights and the formal establishment of ethics committees to assist decision making have helped to formalize the process of ethical decision making in medical care settings. The ethical dilemmas described by the critical care nurses interviewed for this study rarely reflect such a formal decision-making process. Rather, they reveal the perceptions of individuals caught up in the realities of the patient care situation. Making judgments and then deliberately acting on them is essential to the practice of nursing and medicine in hospitals. The decisions made affect the nurses and physicians, their patients, and the institutions and communities where they are located. Responsible decision making usually involves ethical choice but is rarely preceded by the complex and formal deliberation described by Benjamin and Curtis.

Ethical choice in nursing involves issues of accountability, responsibility, and legal definitions of nursing practice. Sigman (1979: 41) has said, "Situations do not present themselves with labels attached. . . . The crux is in the labeling, or the decision . . . depends on how a situation is 'seen.'" Many factors will determine how a situation is "seen." The individual characters of nurses, their gender, race, financial status, and region of birth and personal development, and the nature of their socialization process into nursing education and practice are but a few of these factors. The roles that nurses fulfill in delivering patient care provide another window on the ways in which a situation is "seen."

Elsie and Bertram Bandman (1990: 15–21) have identified the roles that nurses assume with patients that provide the basis for ethical choice.

The nurse-patient relationship fosters the two major roles of surrogate and advocate. The surrogate role implies complete trust, and the nurse is in a position of protecting the patient's most fundamental interests and rights, especially when the patient is helpless. The nurse becomes an agent for the patient in mediating between the patient's interests and the outside world. The nurse may be eyes, ears, arms, legs, and lungs for the patient, compensating for physiological or psychosocial deficits.

The role of advocate implies the protection of the patient's rights. The nurse may accomplish this through other roles such as health educator, technical expert, counselor, leader, or friend. Bandman and Bandman present three arguments rebutting the arguments against nurses as advocates. First, it is sometimes noted, nurses have no institutional protection when acting as patient advocate. Conflicts with physicians and others could cost the nurse his or her job. Bandman and Bandman respond that nurses may be projecting a future role. Patients' rights are in need of protection, and nurses are the logical persons to fulfill this role. Second, some physicians regard themselves as the primary patient advocate and resent intrusion by others. In response, Bandman and Bandman reply that all physicians are not always responsible and accountable. Further, as noted in Chapter 1, critical care nurses are increasingly liable for their own practice (Garlo, 1984). Accountability for co-dependent practice is one aspect of this liability. Third, nurses may assume too many simultaneous roles to have the time, skill, and ability to serve as advocates. Others, for example lawyers, may be better trained for the advocacy role. The rebuttal to this argument is one of the predominant themes stated by critical care nurses. No other group has more continuous contact with patients and families than do nurses. Nurses are often the most familiar with patients' and families' ethical choices and are in a good position to protect those interests in critical care situations.

The professional organizations have formalized codes of ethics. The American Nurses' Association (ANA) code for nurses published in 1976 and revised in 1985 gives eleven precepts addressing issues of patient privacy, respect for human dignity, competence, and a commitment to the public health. Of particular note is a reference to the role of advocate: "The nurse acts to safeguard the client and the public when health care and safety are affected by the incompetent, unethical, or illegal practice of any person" and "the nurse assumes responsibility and accountability for individual nursing judgement and actions" (American Nurses' Association, 1985).

Contemporary medical treatment has produced a changed set of circumstances surrounding death in the hospital setting. Several social trends and shifts have contributed to these changes. People are living longer and are surviving previously fatal diseases to die of something else. Individuals are, in increasing numbers, being treated and dying in hospitals rather than at home. Technology — notably, cardiopulmonary resuscitation (CPR) and equipment and procedures to perform the functions of the vital organs, or to replace the heart, lungs, kidneys, pancreas, liver, and bone marrow — has extended life and death beyond previously defined limits of medical intervention. These same trends have changed both the definition of death and the nature of the care that dying patients receive in hospitals. Both these issues will be explored later in this chapter.

Death was long regarded as a natural and inevitable outcome of illness, disaster, or longevity. Increasingly, as interventions became more successful, death was often postponed or held in abeyance. Since the development of cardiopulmonary resuscitation, a radical shift has occurred in the approach to death in the hospital setting and elsewhere. Surviving illness was once considered the rare occurrence. Death was far more common and regarded as the norm. Since the demonstrated effectiveness of CPR at restoring life, resuscitation is a requirement in hospital settings unless specific orders of "do not resuscitate" (DNR) are arranged for a particular patient. Challenging death has emerged as the norm. Criteria for determining candidates for resuscitation are not clear, although some texts attempt to state criteria such as "all others should be regarded as candidates for resuscitation, except those with known terminal illness and those who have been clinically dead for more than five minutes" (Hudak, Gallo and Lohr, 1990: 94–96). In practice, all hospitalized individuals who die must have CPR initiated, unless a current DNR order has been written by the attending physician after documented consultation with patient, family, or guardian. The Joint Commission on Accreditation of Healthcare Organizations requires that all hospital personnel receive training and review of CPR techniques, at least annually (*AMH 92*, 1992: 80–81).

The changes in intervention for death in hospitals have created great diversity in outcomes for patient prognosis. Successful resuscitation may result in complete recovery, initiation of artificial means of life support in a brain dead individual, or many stages in between. Unsuccessful resuscitation results in death, but a death surrounded by strangers, equipment, and chaos. As these patterns of treatment became universal in American hospitals, they gave rise to many ethical issues, including appropriate levels of intervention and care for DNR patients with regard to diagnostic tests, surgery, administration of blood and antibiotics, and especially feeding and hydration. The dilemmas of achieving death with dignity, or a peaceful, comfortable death, were also exacerbated. Hospitals, as O'Mara (1987: 24) has noted, are increasingly offering patients the opportunity and refining procedures for competent and ethical decision making. Further, various professional groups are attempting to establish codes of ethics and guidelines for intervention with regard to withdrawing or withholding food and fluids (ANA, Committee on Ethics, 1988: 797–800).

Issues related to the right of patients and/or their guardians to make decisions to bring about death with dignity were brought into clear focus by the Nancy Cruzan case. Nancy Cruzan was in a persistent vegatative state following an automobile accident. Her parents successfully petitioned a Missouri court to have her gastrostomy tube removed, but on appeal the Supreme Court of the State of Missouri reversed the decision, citing Cruzan's "right to life." This decision was upheld by the United States Supreme Court, citing a lack of "clear and convincing evidence" of Cruzan's wishes. Further evidence of her wishes was later introduced, her nutrition and hydration were removed, and she died.

The case crystallized legal issues of "right to life," "right to refuse medical treatment," and acceptable "standard of evidence" of a person's wishes (Wurzbach, 1993: 226–230). One of the outcomes of this focused public awareness is the Patient Self-Determination Act (PSDA), enacted by Congress in October 1990 (Omnibus Reconciliation Act, 1990). The act was intended to increase public awareness of health care options and choices, especially advance directives. The PSDA requires all health care institutions that receive federal funds to inform patients of their rights to make decisions about medical treatment, including the right to refuse medical or surgical treatment and the right to formulate advance directives such as a living will and durable power of attorney for health care (Elpern, Yellen, and Burton, 1993: 161–167).

Nurses interviewed for this study expressed a great deal of satisfaction about situations where patients were allowed to die with dignity when death was inevitable (as in brain death or multiple system failure) or appropriate (as in end-stage terminal illness). They expressed considerable frustration about those times when patients were not allowed to die with dignity, as when inappropriate resuscitation or extraordinary treatment was instituted or not withdrawn or when life-support care was continued beyond the patient's request. Communication seemed to be a key issue in these situations. Nurses facilitated communication between patients and families, patients and doctors, and families and doctors. As painful as the losses of dying could be for patients, families, and the medical team, the mechanical support of brain dead patients was worse, and was described as stressful and dehumanizing. Nurses were grateful when decisions were made and treatment plans, developed in conjunction with nursing, medicine, patient, and family, were clear. When technological possibilities dictated the care received, the treatment seemed to assume a life and momentum of its own. Participation in that process was described as devastating. Even in the presence of communication, language often failed. In the presence of hope for life, how can one explain the dehumanizing consequences of treatment?

Terry James speaks of the issues that she sees as related to dying with dignity in the hospital setting:

I think probably one of the most difficult issues that nurses deal with, including myself, is sometimes the right to let the patient die with dignity. Definitely the "no code" issue, definitely the issues where the physicians really do not want the patients coded but yet for whatever reasons they really have not cleared that with the patient or the family to the point that they would write the order to legally cover you for not taking any action should the patient succumb. I think that invasion of privacy on the part of the patient is an issue, and I think sometimes the dehumanization of the patient is also an issue.

What are you thinking about when you talk about invasion of privacy and dehumanization?

I think that a lot of times that we are all very guilty of, particularly for your more acute patients who cannot verbalize, talking over the patient and about the patient, giving very little regard to what the patient is hearing, what the patient is interpreting, and, subsequently, what he's feeling about the conversation.

What about privacy?

I think that there are a lot of times when it's really easy to go into a patient's room and to do something to them and for them and it's such a matter of routine that it's easy to forget to do things like to shut the door, close the venetian blinds, that kind of thing.

What ethical decisions have you made or have you seen made in ICU by nurses and colleagues?

I have seen where nurses have been approached by physicians who for whatever reasons would not write the "no code" orders and asked to *not* call a code, and when something happens to the patient, then the nurses call the code. I think nurses have stood their ground about that, and I think that many times they have been fussed at by physicians for doing that, because that is not what the physician desired but that's the way it had to be. The physician had not written the order. I think, too, that nurses have felt more comfortable communicating to physicians when patients or families express their desire in terms of the "no code."

Say that again?

When patients and families have been open in discussing the "no code" issues with the nurses more than to the physicians, and in turn, the physicians have not been as open to the patients and families, then I think the nurses have taken more of a stand to approach physicians and say, "Look . . . !"

Nurses actively communicate between the family, the patient, and the physician?

Yes.

Can you think of other ethical situations?

I think, yeah, I think that when there are situations where the interaction between physicians and patient is less than desirable that nurses have addressed that, they've confronted it, and if need be they have reported it to folks who could take care of it. I think that nurses have been an advocate as far as making sure that the patients were informed and that when a doctor flips in and says, "Hi, I'm going to do your open heart surgery tomorrow, see you later," and the patient's anxiety level has gone out the roof, he's got a lot of questions and concerns. Then again the nurse has served as the one who would get physicians, whomever, to come in and talk to the patient and kind of get their questions answered.

Has the appearance of AIDS presented some ethical dilemmas for you or your staff?

I don't think so. We have not had a lot of patients with AIDS and in fact I can only think of one that we had who died because of AIDS, one who died that we didn't even know that he had AIDS at the time he died, and I think that in those situations that the nurses were more concerned about transmission, being careful about blood and that kind of thing, than any ethical issues per se.

Is it difficult for nurses? Are nurses afraid of those patients?

I don't think that nurses are necessarily as afraid of the patients as they are careful with the patients. But I think, in my unit in particular, we have had so many patients with so many unusual contagious, communicable kinds of things that all of the nurses are careful with all the patients, and one of the things that I stress in the unit is do not practice under the philosophy, "If I had only known I would have been more careful." We treat everyone as if they had the worst communicable disease in the world.

Advocacy was identified as a major role in the care of dying patients by Margie Goodrum:

Are there ethical decisions that nurses make?

Well, we are involved in all of these decisions. As patient advocates, we have to be involved in all the technology. We can't control who is admitted, but we can protest inappropriate admissions into ICU. We get people out when it is not appropriate, and we do question as patient advocates. I have often done this when patients have told me, "I don't know why he is giving me these tests." I have told them that they have the right to (a) not have the test done and (b) most importantly, to have the physician explain to you why he thinks it is necessary to have this test done. If you can't see why it is necessary, then you don't have to have it done. I think this is educating patients and that they have a right. This is their body and they have a say in it. That is a very important ethical issue that nurses get into.

You just don't go up to somebody and say, "Your doctor isn't really competent." But patients will ask you, "Do you think this is appropriate? Do you think I need this?" I try to explain it. Sometimes I go back to the chart and look at the doctor's progress notes. Or I will talk to the doctor and ask why he wants to do this test or try to find out some information for the patient. I never say, "This is absurd." I say, "I don't know the reason he wants to do it. I can't really find his basis for deciding this in the chart, but I think that you need to understand why you need to have this test done before you have it done, and he should explain to you what it is that he is looking to find and why he thinks it is necessary. If you don't think that he has come up with a good reason then you don't have to have this test done. This is your option."

Then, there are other times when patients refuse treatments that I may feel are necessary, and I will talk to the doctor to find out what is going on and why they are refusing. I think patients have a right to decide that, but I think that you need to make sure that they have the knowledge to make that decision. It is still their decision, and I would not make anybody do anything, but I will try to find out what is going on and give them information that is needed.

So nurses do intervene in these kinds of situations?

Absolutely, because a lot of times patients will express doubts to us or ask us questions if they don't ask the doctor. We are a lot more accessible. We are with them a lot more. We are not seen as being in a hurry, and doctors are. "He breezes in and out of here, and he is always in a hurry. I never can think of things when he is in here because he is only in here for a few minutes." I tell them, "Write it down. Have a list. Tell him you have got some questions and if he can't talk to you now he can come back in a few hours when he has got time, but you are going to ask him these questions." You have to teach patients to be assertive with their doctors so that they can get the care that they deserve.

In a difficult situation, you mentioned peaceful death being hard in a hospital. What is difficult for the nurse about those situations?

Because we are the ones that do the stuff. We are the ones who are doing it. We are the ones who are dealing with a dying person who is not allowed to die peacefully. He is always being poked and prodded and things kept going artificially. And you are the one who is there with them. The doctor walks in, but he doesn't stay with them. You are the one who has to deal with it. You are the one who is there. You are the one to whom the family is saying, "But I don't understand. What is happening?"

Or it may be the patient whom you feel like is a victim. The nurse is always there and it is always harder on the nurse. The doctor can leave the unit. The doctor is not the one who usually initiates treatment. A lot of ethical decisions come by default to nurses. We are the ones who are there. If the doctor doesn't write "no code," then it is our decision in initiating the code, which is not really a decision because legally you have to initiate a code. There are codes that are run a little less rapidly than other codes. It is a fact of life. If you don't feel like somebody should be coded, it's, "All right, we are going to start this code, but you go ahead and call the medical house officer or call the attending [physician] because he can stop it." That kind of thing instead of, "Gee, let's jump on it!"

I also think that pain is an ethical issue. Getting something ordered for patients. Pain can be a problem. You can't get an order or nurses are hesitant to give it for fear of depressing someone's respiration. Providing pain medication when somebody is in pain, but unstable, is also an ethical issue. Pain medication usually has an effect on that instability, depressing either the respiratory or cardiovascular system. That can be a real dilemma. Usually you have to be the judge of what to give and how much to give. Patients' rights. Consent forms. Nurses are involved in all of it.

Margie Goodrum describes the frustrations of another situation, when the nurses and the patient were caught in a crisis of indecision. A "no code" or "don't resuscitate" decision must be made by the primary attending physician in consultation with the patient or family. This decision is made when there is no hope of recovery or appropriate intervention. Hopefully, a patient who is not competent will have a living will or a person designated as having durable power of attorney for health care to direct this decision. If an order is not written, hospital staff are obligated to resuscitate. These patients often end up mechanically ventilated and unresponsive. Even if they are not comatose, they can no longer speak because of the breathing tube.

We have had a lot of patients that, since the attending physician has to write the "no code" order, you can't get a "no code" order, and it has just been a crime, and you just pray that they don't code until you can get the "no code" order from that physician. It is just a crime what we do. Working weekends is just real frustrating because the physician who admitted them is off and his partner is on and he won't make a decision. "Well, he will make a decision on Monday morning." Well, in the meantime this patient is an inch away from coding. We had this one lady who had toxic epidural necrolysis [massive allergic response to antibiotics or other drugs], and she was sloughing off her skin. She also had DIC [disseminating intravascular coagulation], and she was bleeding all over the place. A little old Black lady. She was the most pitiful thing that I had ever seen in my whole entire life. She was lying in this fluid-filled bed. We were literally suctioning her bed out because there was so much blood that she just constantly oozed. She was wet all over like she had been burned. We could not get a "no code" on this lady the whole damned weekend. It was one of the most frustrating things that I had ever dealt with. The attending physician was not on call, and his partner would not make a decision, would not even come in and see her. The residents were well aware of this, because we made them well aware. The residents on the service and also the resident who was the medical house officer, we just made them well aware. We said, "All right, when she goes you will be up here, and you will call the attending and we will stop it immediately." It would have been a crime. In the first place, you could not have defibrillated her because she was constantly lying in a pool of blood because there was nothing that we could do to keep her dry. I literally suctioned her bed out hourly.

Was she alert?

She was comatose by this time, thank God. She had been worked on for a long time. She had been in the unit for a while and had just gotten worse and worse, and they just could not get it to turn around. She had a lot of problems. But the lady, I was so proud of her, she coded [heart stopped beating—cardiac *arrest] Monday morning at nine A.M. when her attending was in the unit, so she did not get coded because he made her a "no code" at that time.*

Nurses expressed much satisfaction when patients who had no hope of recovery to good quality of life were allowed to die with dignity. Similarly, much frustration was felt about participation in situations where extraordinary treatments were continued on patients who had no reasonable expectation of recovery. Nurses perceived these forms of treatment as cruelty and torture. Inappropriate CPR and resuscitation, initiating or refusing to withdraw extraordinary means of care (drugs, ventilator, diagnostic tests), or life support continued beyond the patient's request are examples of those kinds of treatments. Often the most difficult periods occurred prior to the decisions made about DNR orders. Physicians and family often postponed this decision-making process.

Death with dignity was accomplished through clear communication and consensus about treatment among patients, family, physicians, and the nursing staff. Nurses believed they were especially effective at facilitating this communication for several key reasons. First, nurses are personally involved and heavily invested both emotionally and physically in the patient's care, and effective decision making reduces the pain and conflict in the situation. Nurses are there "doing the stuff" and inflicting "pain" and "torture" against patients' best interests or their wishes. Second, nurses are accessible continuously to patients and families, while physicians are there for limited periods. Nurses may sense when a patient is tired and decisions need to be made. They also may help identify resources within a family unit to assist in the grief process. Third, nurses believed that patients confided secrets to them that they were unable to share with the family or the physician. Nurses felt that patients trusted the nurse to act as advocate, in the patient's behalf, to initiate the process of decision making to achieve the DNR orders or withdrawal of treatment that would enable them to have a peaceful death.

Richard Pate, thirty-four, a critical care nurse for eight years, beginning in 1979, and the only male in the sample, speaks of the ethical dilemmas he has experienced in practice:

What do you think are the ethical dilemmas that you see with patient care that you have experienced?

Keeping people alive who do not want to be kept alive. And I think that has changed also. Now I am a person who has taken a number of people off ventilators. I've never felt the least bit of compunction or moral indecision about that. The worst experiences I ever had was a woman who had had open heart surgery and developed TEN [toxic epidermal necrolysis] from Dilantin [a drug for seizures], I believe it was in her case. Anyway, she was horribly ill, and one day I was working on one of her major wounds in the neuro ICU, and she looked at me and said, "Why are you doing this to me? You know I'm going to die." And I did. And so did everybody else. And yet we tortured her for an additional six weeks. That was—that is an ethical dilemma, and we're seeing a lot less of it now.

You said you had been in the position to take people off ventilators.

Well, in the neuro ICU, of course. You know a lot of brain death occurs there, as in any neurosurgical setting—those people we took off ventilators. I actually took off the ventilator the "first right to die case" in Georgia, who was a gentleman with ALS [amyotrophic lateral sclerosis] who had been maintained at home for eight years. And he was, of course, of perfectly sound intellect. And he had always said that if he ever became ventilator-dependent, he would want to be taken off the vent. And he did become ventilator-dependent. We just could not get him off. And his wife and the head nurse went to petition a DeKalb County Superior Court judge, who came to the hospital, took a deposition from the patient, went back to his office, and wrote a restraining order prohibiting us from delivering any further medical assistance. And so I gave him a hundred milligrams of IV [intravenous] Demerol and extubated him [removed the breathing tube]. And he died. And it was the most touching thing I'd ever seen. It was his wife, who obviously loved him more than anything, fulfilling his last and absolutely necessary wish. It was truly lovely. And, you know, I was happy to do it. The ethical decision I have to make is continuing to work on someone when it's obvious that either they will not live or that their quality of life will be so horribly sub-optimum.

Do you feel like you're basically powerless in those situations?

I think that we all have options. Whether or not we choose to exercise them is quite another story. I engage physicians in conversation about—how far do we go? I have suggested that it's time to stop, and I feel perfectly free to do that. I think ultimately the one person with responsibility over a patient's care is the attending physician. Everyone else just adds to it. Even the consulting physicians don't write orders. They recommend things, so I don't feel any more powerless than anyone else in that situation. I think that's an inherent part of the medical system that has the ability to keep people alive who would not otherwise be alive. Particularly with respiration.

Pate makes several succinct points. The nurse is a skilled member of a team and is obligated to be vocal. The dilemmas experienced by nurses in those situations are also felt by physicians. And the legal system has begun to reflect some of the social changes that have occurred as a result of rapid changes in life support technologies. The rights of patients to die with dignity when no hope exists of return to an acceptable quality of life are more and more protected. Another factor that has altered the entire medical and legal arena in the death with dignity issue is the evolution of the definition of death from the traditional cessation of heartbeat and breathing to the current one of brain death and/or documented persistent poor prognosis. The evolution of this definition was certainly influenced by both the use of the ventilator and the successful transplant of human organs and tissues.

Early respirators were used in the treatment of patients with polio and with near-drowning victims. After the 1950s, more refined ventilators were used successfully for temporary support after neurosurgery, cardiac surgery, myocardial infarction, and drug overdose. This technology has reduced mortality and is a useful tool. Ventilators are becoming increasingly common in both large urban hospitals and small rural ones. Since ventilators are as common in the long-term support of patients with multiple complications as they are in short-term crisis management, the problems associated with their use are more evident. The respirator can ventilate individuals who could not breathe on their own and who might also have loss of brain function. A person can "live" on the machine until death occurs from heart failure, infection, or some other cause. The dilemma of removing life-support technology is as problematic as initiating it. Because the technology exists, hospitals, nurses, and physicians are obligated to initiate life-supportive, resuscitative efforts when a patient dies unless prior advisement with the patient and/or family and legal action have allowed a "do not resuscitate" order to be written. Hospitalized patients, even if terminally ill, are at the mercy of the technology, especially if a medical crisis or death occurs very quickly. Certainly long-term ventilator support has helped many persons to survive with good quality of life. The expense of such treatments and the dilemmas in decision making do not influence either the realities of initiating treatment or the likelihood of success or failure as outcome. The technology exists and is used.

"Death," ethicist Robert Veatch observes, "has always been inevitable. Where humans were once helpless observers in the presence of death, we are increasingly able to intervene in the process, using technological resources to direct or delay the inevitable" (Veatch, 1977: 2–3). His observation seems to reflect humanity's struggle against death in the presence of ambivalence and fear. Paul Ramsey has described the role of contemporary health care personnel in this context: "The conviction that one should always choose life lies at the heart of the practice of medicine and nursing. Medical ethics must be pro-life in this context. This aspect of modern medicine was profoundly influenced by Judaism and Christianity" (Ramsey, 1978: 146–147). The mandate to "choose life" appears absolute and definitive, yet no clarification is offered on the meaning of either quality of life or good and peaceful death. American society, in particular, denies death and conspires to keep it hidden from view. Modern funeral practices demonstrate this. The denial of death is focused in situations where death occurs in hospital settings, where technology is available to keep death at abeyance indefinitely. As G. H. Kieffer notes, "Death has been transformed from 'God's will' to a 'natural event' to an 'untimely event'" (Kieffer, 1979: 214–215).

The ventilator and artificial nutrition and hydration, either by a feeding tube into the stomach or bowel or by an intravenous line, have made extraordinary means of life support possible. Issues related to withdrawing or withholding food and fluids continue to be special problems for nurses, particularly in the care of severely handicapped newborns or patients with documented brain death. The issues are not completely identified or articulated, but efforts are underway by nurses, ethicists, legal advisors, consumers, and others to continue compassionate clarification of the human rights issues involved (ANA Committee on Ethics, 1988: 797–801; Martin, 1985: 47–56).

Concerns about artificial prolongation of the dying process, in many dying or critically ill patients or patients who are alert or who have made advance directives, have generated a debate about the issues involved in withdrawing or withholding artificial nutrition and hydration. L. S. Knox (1989: 427–436) and M. E. Wurzbach (1990: 226–230) provide current literature and case review and sensitive discussions of these issues. The debate between humanitarian life extension and comfort versus selective withdrawal of nutrition and hydration will likely continue for some time. Certainly, critical care nurses are participants at the center of this debate. Similar concerns have emerged related to the withdrawal of mechanical ventilator support. Guidelines for terminal weaning and the ethical issues involved with goals for patient and family comfort are discussed in the recent literature (AACN, 1990; Campbell and Carlson, 1992: 52–56; Daly et al., 1993: 217–223).

The fourth edition of *Black's Law Dictionary,* published in 1968, reflected the traditional definition of death as "the cessation of life, the ceasing to exist, defined by physicians as a total stoppage of the circulation of the blood, and a cessation of the animal and vital functions consequent thereupon, such as respiration, pulsation, etc." (Black, 1968; Wojcik, 1978: 95). Machines that ventilate and circulate a body nourished by artificial means have rendered this definition meaningless. Technology created a semblance of life that must be distinguished from traditionally understood and valued styles of life and death. William May has articulated the problem well. "In the service of saving life," May writes, "heroic medicine can sometimes only assure that its final moments will be as miserable as possible. Humanity is tested in the way we behave toward death . . . and it is obscured and diminished when death is concealed from view, . . . when the dying are forced to make their exit anonymously, their ending unwitnessed, uncherished, and unrecorded except in the hospital files" (May, 1972: 488).

By the end of the 1970s, sophisticated intensive care units became commonplace in hospitals, and the possibilities of sustaining circulation and breathing, equated with "life," were a reality for almost all hospital patients. In the early 1980s, rapid pharmacological advances in immunosuppressant drug therapy precipitated a rapid emergence of organ transplant surgery. The capacity for successful organ transplant, and media attention to organ procurement and recipient issues, soon brought into focus the problems of traditional definitions of death, which were seen as obsolete (Ufford, 1986). A donor organ had to be maintained by adequate circulation until transport to the recipient is initiated. If pronouncement of death in a donor was delayed until the heart or lungs stopped functioning, the life-saving transplant surgery could be jeopardized by deterioration of the donor organs. On the other hand, by the traditional definition of death, removal of vital organs before the heart and lungs failed constituted murder. These dilemmas illustrate the complexities involved and the need for a clear definition of death based on brain function.

Many cases were cited that documented the need for brain death legislation. A victim of a gunshot wound to the head provides an example. The "brain dead" patient was not pronounced dead by the physician until after the heart had stopped beating. The defendant, charged with murder, claimed that the patient did not die from a gunshot wound to the head (which had resulted in his brain death) but rather that the doctors had caused his death by removing his life support systems (O'Hara, 1982: 109). The case of *Tucker versus Lower* illustrates the issues involved with organ transplant.

The case involved a $1,000,000 wrongful death action against four physicians. The decedent's brother alleged that removal of the heart for transplantation was begun before the donor's death, that is, while vital functions were being maintained by mechanical means. Defendants argued that the donor was dead at the time of excision, since an encephalogram indicated that he had experienced cerebral death and had been incapable of spontaneous respiration for a period of five minutes. At the beginning of the trial the judge felt that until the Virginia legislature interceded, the common-law definition of death must apply. By the end of the trial, after hearing extensive medical testimony on brain death, he charged the jury: " . . . you shall determine the time of death in this case by using the following definition of the nature of death. Death is a cessation of life. It is the ceasing to exist. Under the law, death is not continuing but occurs at a precise time. . . . In determining . . . you may consider the following elements . . . among them, the time of complete and irreversible loss of all function of the brain." The jury returned in 77 minutes with a verdict in favor of the defendant physicians. (*Tucker v. Lower,* 1972)

Attempts to determine both criteria for the use of extraordinary means of life support and a meaningful definition of death have both clarified and confused the issue. Furthermore, the changes in common understanding of the meaning of a natural death, and increasing demands by individuals for choice, have generated litigation and policy changes, such as the Karen Ann Quinlan case and the brain death determination statutes in various states. Karen Ann Quinlan, in a deep coma, but not brain dead, after a drug overdose, was removed from the ventilator after her parents, on her behalf, petitioned the courts and then appealed to the New Jersey Supreme Court, to protect her privacy and allow her to die with dignity. She lived for several years in a vegetative state, fed through a nasogastric feeding tube but breathing on her own. The lower court prohibited the withdrawal of the respirator, determining that since there is no constitutional right to die, the withdrawal of life support is murder. The New Jersey Supreme Court overturned the lower court's ruling. In its decision, the major concern was the violation of Quinlan's right to privacy: "We think that the state's interest contra weakens and the individual's right to privacy grow as the degree of bodily invasion increases and the prognosis dims" (*Matter of Quinlan,* 1976). This landmark case established a precedent for removal of artificial life-support measures in the presence of brain death (Bandman and Bandman, 1990: 57; *In re Quinlan,* 1975).

In 1957, Pope Pius XII attempted to deal with the morality of resuscitation in a public statement:

Man . . . has a duty to preserve life and health, but is obliged to use only ordinary means to achieve this end—those which do not impose ponderous hardships on oneself or on others. Ordinary means signify those in keeping with the circumstances of the person, place, time, and culture. Physicians are not obligated to use extraordinary means—specifically modern respiratory technology—in cases "considered to be completely hopeless" by the physician and when the treatment would go against the wishes of the family. (Pius XII, 1958: 393)

While this statement clarifies criteria for use of extraordinary means, it neither defines what is ordinary nor prescribes moral action if a person is already attached to a respirator when the hopeless state occurs. Value judgments on what defines quality of life for the aged, the terminally ill, the hopelessly malformed neonate, or the functionally dead remain obscure. These value judgments become even more complex if the body attached to the ventilator has an organ or body part suitable for transplantation or if the critical care bed is needed for another patient with more hope for recovery to a conscious and independent state. This debate will continue (McCaman, 1976; Stein, 1978; Ufford, 1986).

In 1968, an Ad Hoc Committee of the Harvard Medical School published a report entitled "A Definition of Irreversible Coma." This document was widely criticized and defended, and ultimately accepted by most medical practitioners, as it does provide specific parameters in the definition of death. The report lists four criteria:

1. Unreceptivity and unresponsivity: total unawareness of externally applied stimuli and complete unresponsiveness to even the most intensely painful stimuli (no vocal or other response such as a groan, withdrawal of a limb, quickening of respiration).

2. Movements or breathing: no spontaneous muscular movements or response to any stimuli (pain, light, sound, touch), or spontaneous respiration; both of the above should not be observed covering a period of one hour. After patient is on a mechanical respirator, the total absence of spontaneous breathing is tested by turning off the respirator for three minutes and observing whether any effort to breathe spontaneously is made.

3. No reflexes: pupils fixed and dilated and do not respond to bright light; no ocular movements to head turning or following irrigation of ears with ice water, and no blinking; no evidence of postural activity; corneal and pharyngeal reflexes absent; no swallowing, yawning, or vocalization reflexes; no motor reflexes whatsoever (biceps, triceps, pronator muscles, quadriceps, and gastrocnemius); all of the above indicative of irreversible coma.

4. Flat electroencephalogram: isoelectric or flat EEG; at least a full ten minutes of recordings. This is confirmatory only; not diagnostic. (Kieffer, 1979: 213)

These tests repeated 24 hours later should reveal no change. If the repeat still reveals no activity, then the patient can be judged dead on the basis of irreversible cerebral damage (Ad Hoc Committee of the Harvard Medical School, 1968: 337–340; Beauchamp and Walter, 1989: 142–153; Black, 1990: 188; Davis and Aroskar, 1991: 142–145; Kieffer, 1979: 213).·

The Task Force on Death and Dying of the Institute of Society, Ethics and Life Sciences, in evaluating the Harvard criteria, voiced four areas of concern: the vagueness of the definition of death (the criteria assert that death has occurred, but not precisely when it has occurred); the fear that the new criteria are primarily intended to facilitate transplants; mistrust of new powers vested in the attending physician; and fears that the new definition will lend itself to updating at an increasing risk to the dignity of the dying patient (Wojcik, 1978: 100). Significantly, the Harvard criteria address only the definition of patient death, not when treatment should be withdrawn to allow the patient to die or when treatment should not be initiated.

The Harvard criteria for determining brain death or irreversible coma were soon validated in 1974 by the Royal College of the United Kingdom and in 1977 by further studies that established the credibility of the Harvard study findings (Appraisal Criteria, 1977; Slemanda, 1983). In the United States, individual states began, in 1971, to initiate brain death legislation. Since Kansas enacted the first statute in 1971, at least 25 states have passed brain death statutes with wide variance in language. The trend toward a uniform brain death statute was solidified by the independent adoption, in 1979, of a model statute, the Uniform Brain Death Act, prepared by the American Bar Association, the American Medical Association and the National Conference of Commissioners on Uniform State Laws (O'Hara, 1982). This model statute, the Uniform Determination of Death Act, was endorsed by the President's Commission for the Study of Ethical Problems in Medicine and Biomedical and Behavioral Research, the American Academy of Neurology, and the American Electroencephalographic Society. Rather than stating explicit diagnostic criteria that might change with new technology, the statute supports the application of accepted medical standards for determining brain death. The statute reads, "An individual who has sustained either (1) irreversible cessation of circulatory and respiratory functions, or (2) irreversible cessation of all functions of the entire brain, including the brain stem, is dead. A determination of death must be made in accordance with acceptable medical standards" (O'Hara, 1982; Ufford, 1986). This act is adopted by most states at the present time.

Determination of brain death usually requires the independent assessment of another physician. The fifth edition of *Black's Law Dictionary* (Black, 1979: 170) states the following definition of brain death: "A person shall be pronounced dead if it is determined by a physician that the person has suffered a total and irreversible cessation of brain function. There shall be independent confirmation of the death by another physician." The Harvard criteria provide the basis for determining brain death. By the time that the sixth edition of *Black's Law Dictionary* was published, the definition of brain death closely modeled the Uniform Determination of Death Act and the Harvard criteria: "Characteristics of brain death consist of: (1) unreceptivity and unresponsiveness to externally applied stimuli and internal needs; (2) no spontaneous movements or breathing; (3) no reflex activity; and (4) a flat electroencephalographic reading after 24 hour period of observation" (Black, 1990: 188).

"Do not resuscitate" (DNR) orders, also referred to as "no code," are the source of much controversy for nurses and others caring for critically ill patients in hospitals. These patients may have a terminal illness, brain death, or a health status that is complex, complicated, and progressive in deterioration and hopelessness. A DNR order essentially means that cardiopulmonary resuscitative measures will be withheld in the event of acute cardiac or respiratory arrest (Miles, Cranford, and Schultz, 1982). Given this definition, other forms of life-sustaining interventions such as antibiotics, feeding and hydration, and blood products can be and are administered to patients with DNR orders. In critical care units especially, where lifesaving technology is commonplace, decisions often must be made about which specific treatments should be initiated, withheld, or discontinued.

Lewandowski et al. (1985: 175–181) note that health professionals, families, and patients often disagree about the type and level of treatment to be provided to DNR patients. Attitudes range between two extremes, from the view that, except for CPR, all aggressive medical and nursing activities will be continued or initiated to the perspective that DNR patients should be allowed to die quietly and with dignity, a view that implies the withdrawal of life-sustaining medical intervention and the provision of only comfort measures. The researchers designed a study to examine the following three questions about DNR patients in a medical ICU. What levels of medical and nursing resources are consumed by DNR patients in the ICU? What is the impact of the DNR order and the withdrawal or initiation of life-saving and nursing interventions? Do DNR patients survive the ICU and hospital? A group of 506 patients admitted for one year to a medical ICU in an urban northern city were studied. Of these patients 71 were designated DNR during their hospital stay and none of the DNR orders were rescinded during the stay in the ICU. Of the DNR patients, 55 (77%) died in the ICU and another seven died on the medical ward after transfer from the ICU. Nine of the 71 patients lived and were discharged from the hospital. The mortality rate for the entire ICU population for the year was 17 percent.

The researchers examined resource consumption and nursing care requirements of both DNR and non-DNR patients in the ICU. Life-saving interventions, including ventilators, vasopressors, anti-arrhythmics, intravenous antibiotics, and pulmonary artery catheters, were continued on 73 percent of the patients who had them before the DNR order was written. A high percentage (91%) of ventilated patients remained on ventilators after being designated DNR. With the exception of ventilators, other treatments and diagnostic procedures (bronchoscopy, sigmoidoscopy, and abdominal ultrasound) were initiated on patients after DNR orders were written.

Nursing care requirements showed a similar trend. DNR patients required more nursing care than all other non-DNR patients, including those non-DNR patients who were seriously ill. A DNR designation did not alter the amount of nursing care required. DNR patients continued to have intense physical dependency needs and moderate to high social and emotional needs after the DNR order was written. Minimal rehabilitation and teaching were required both before and after the DNR order. The level of required observation decreased after the DNR order, although this reduced level was still assessed as being in the high to intense range.

The findings provide needed data both about the characteristics and treatment of DNR patients in a critical care setting and about the ambiguities involved in the meaning of the DNR order to patients, families, and health care personnel. The study reveals the following findings. It was common for DNR patients to occupy beds in an MICU (medical intensive care unit). Decisions about DNR designation and the appropriateness of varied levels of patient care were common issues in the critical care setting. DNR patients had very long ICU stays and consumed equal or greater medical and nursing resources than patients who were candidates for resuscitation. Patients who were DNR on the ward were transferred to the

ICU. In fact, a DNR order was neither an indication that the physicians and nurses stopped caring for the patient nor a mandate for transfer out of the ICU.

Further, DNR patients continued to receive aggressive treatment. Although ventilation was not initiated after the DNR order, it was not withdrawn. Despite grave prognoses, physicians continued to treat DNR patients aggressively. Despite this level of intervention, the mortality rate remained very high. The issues of withdrawal of medical treatment and questions related to the most appropriate care for DNR patients remain largely unaddressed. Is an ICU the appropriate place for nurses to best meet the DNR patient's physical, psychological, and social needs? The researchers note the need for further studies to determine appropriate treatment and care of DNR patients. Continuation of aggressive medical treatment in a patient for whom resuscitation would mean a postponement of death wastes scarce ICU resources and causes undue patient suffering and crippling financial burdens for patients, families, and society. Finally, the researchers advise that future research be focused on the quality of life of DNR patients who survive hospitalization to determine the moral implications of treatment of DNR patients in the hospital setting (Lewandowski et al., 1985: 175–181).

Tittle, Moody, and Becker (1991: 140–144) studied DNR and non-DNR patients in order to identify which variables are the best predictors of a DNR classification so that a model could be developed to predict the level of nursing care required by DNR patients in the ICU. One model identified the best predictor as the origin of admission and the severity of illness on the admission day. A second model identified the best predictor as the number of days spent in the ICU prior to the DNR order, the average daily resource allocation points after the DNR order, and the severity of illness scores on the day the DNR order was designated.

Jezewski et al. (1993: 302–309) studied self-reporting of 22 critical care nurses with at least one year of experience in a critical care unit to investigate the process of consenting to "do not resuscitate" status. A theoretical model was developed that considered issues of timing, the meaning of DNR to family members, areas of conflict, and the role of the nurse, including on-going support of the patient and family.

These studies illustrate the ambiguities involved in treating very ill patients in critical care settings. Nurses are present continuously with these patients and their families during the duration of their ICU and hospital stays. The range of stresses, satisfactions, and frustrations that nurses experience in caring for patients for whom they perceive ethical dimensions of care are well expressed in the following interview data.

Alice Walker describes experiences with brain dead children during a time when the definition of death was in transition. Her reflections provide insight into the experiences and feelings of nurses, physicians, and family members caught up in these situations. Her story also points out the assertive role that a nurse manager can play in bringing about change:

We had a big, big problem with brain death one summer. It was during the time period when those seventeen nurses had come. They didn't all come at one time. They came through the course of a whole summer and seven of them were new graduates. By July they were all in tears and devastated because we had four brain dead patients at one time, out of eight kids. One was a trauma that was a drowning. One was a meningitis. One was an anesthesia accident in the OR [operating room]. And one was also meningitis. So one particular week they were all there at the same time. This is what had happened. The anesthesia accident came in first. They had not hooked up the PEEP valve or something on the ventilator in the OR. And it had been surgery for a hairy nevus or something. It was a real minor kind of procedure, and this child ended up brain dead—an infant, like an eight-month-old. So you had this kid in one bed and next to him you had a meningitis who had been very misdiagnosed at another hospital and had herniated his brain stem before he even got to our hospital and had been basically brain dead since his admission. And then an . . . I forgot what happened to the fourth one—the drowning kid. And so what happened is these other kids are being supported for twenty days on the ventilator, and every day the parents would be told by the attending physician that . . . they had less than a one percent chance of survival. I mean, they were brain dead. They'd been documented everywhere, but they were too afraid to tell them that because—especially of the anesthesia accident—that it was a legal case. So they never really told the parents the truth. They never said the words brain dead—nothing. Just in a coma. Those two were on the medical service because, even that other kid who was an anesthesia problem, he was still on the medical service for some reason. So the neurosurgeon covered the drowning accident one because he ended up coming in and having a craniotomy done because he'd been hit by a boat—not just a drowning, but it was a trauma at the same time, and so that child was diagnosed and taken off the ventilator as brain dead within thirty-six hours and the family was well prepared. The whole thing just went like clockwork. Very smooth. Everybody understood. It was sad, but it was different than these other two cases. So then you have these three cases there together and the new nurses just being up in arms over the whole ethical issue of what was going on and furious about it.

So I finally went that next week—I'd talked to the attendings on the other two kids forever and they wouldn't back down. They said, well, you can't diagnose brain death in children. It's not possible, so we can't say anything. It doesn't matter—and we had a brain death committee in the hospital for adults, but they wouldn't apply to kids. So I went to see this neurosurgeon and said, "You know, okay, if they won't diagnose it brain death, how come you can do it?" And said, "it's just an ongoing battle. There's nothing I can do about it. I've talked to them. It is legal." He gave me a copy of the statute right out of his office. He told me to call the brain death committee people and talk to the chair because he was a neuropsychiatrist. He was also the chairman of the EEG lab. So he was just not your routine psychiatrist. He knew a lot of neuro medicine too. So he told me to go talk to him and that if he could help me in any way he would, but as far as getting these attendings to change their minds, it was like talking to a brick wall. So we ended up working it out to where we got the lawyers to come talk to the doctors and set up a major educational conference for them and rewrote the whole brain death policy for pediatrics so that we could have a system like this neurosurgeon used. But it took about five months to do it. And by that time the other two kids ended up dying before they ever intervened—they never turned them off the ventilator at all and wouldn't back down. But we ended up getting a real positive experience because of working through the surgeon who had a different system—So that also built my confidence in working with attending physicians because I was out to get this problem solved and ended up using somebody that normally I would never have gone to just to talk to, but seeing how he handled things so differently than the other doctors there had to be something to it, and I didn't know any of the legal jargon or any of that stuff until I got "gung ho" on this problem and it ended up wonderfully because we didn't lose any of those nurses. But they were all ready to leave.

"You know," they said, "if this is going to keep happening, we can't handle this." Because it was like lying to the parents. They understood the diagnosis of brain death, because they'd just gotten out of nursing school. But it was a new diagnosis that I think changed a lot of how we're dealing with critical care today. Because the old definition of death was cardiac death and that was one experience I'd had as a first-year nurse in that old hospital. They made me take this little baby down the hall to another room, bagging it with an Ambu bag [breathing for the baby with a manual bag], because we took it off the ventilator and it had herniated and been brain dead probably for about three days—a little two-month-old infant. I had to sit in that room with the baby until his heart stopped, so I could come tell the doctor when to come pronounce him dead. Hours. I had to sit in there like three hours with this baby, and it was a horrible experience. And I didn't understand, you know, all the stuff that was going on because I'd also been taught that heart and respirations was the definition of death. So I understood why they were waiting to pronounce him dead at the time, but that changed in the next two years after that because this was in 1980. And by about 1982 was when the definition of death changed, after the 1981 President's Commission. So that happened to me before the law really did change. But then you have got all these doctors who have been educated even more so than me on pronouncing cardiac death, and you couldn't tell them to change the way they've been taught. They didn't—they understood it, you know, intellectually, but they wouldn't change. Because they were afraid of getting sued, number one.

What gave them the confidence to change?

Seeing on paper that it was legal to do it, for one—and hearing it from the lawyers because they had a big group of lawyers that came and talked to them. And then getting the neurologists and neurosurgeons to set down guidelines for how to make a systematic diagnosis where you'd have things that would cross prove each other over about a 36-hour period, and we couldn't get everybody to agree on the neonates, less than 28 days old you don't know what their brain function is. So we made the time periods for diagnosis longer for the neonates, a moderate amount for the infant and toddler, and then the pre-school-aged child was another one, and over age twelve we treated with the adult criteria. So we had it in four phases like that. Then the physicians were comfortable because they had a list—it was almost like a checklist—they knew that you had to have six tests if it was a newborn, so you'd be doubly sure it was the right diagnosis.

Walker describes patient care situations that reflect the appeal of pediatric ICU care as well as the reality of that care:

So what has been appealing to you about the critical care or intensive care experience with children?

Well, once I stayed in it for awhile—every time somebody would find out where I worked, they'd say, "How can you stand to work with little sick kids in the intensive care unit?" I never looked at it that way because we probably ended up having about a 50/50 mortality/survival rate. Some of the kids did not do well at all. They may have gotten out of the intensive care unit, but they did not do well, and you knew when they left they weren't going to. And then the other 50 percent did great and they were fine and you could see them go from being very, very sick to getting well. Because we did have at least five to six deaths a month usually in the course of a year. We had a fair number, but at the same time those were usually the kinds that were—that hope for survival was real low usually. It usually was not the kids who shouldn't have died. And you could kind of end up rationalizing a lot of that in your mind. And we had two or three patients that I was real, real close to that no one had any idea what was wrong with them. We supported them for two or three weeks on massive amounts of drips and ventilatory support, and they recovered without one problem at all. We called this one kid our miracle baby, and he ended up having a folic acid deficiency from drinking goat's milk that had caused all his metabolic goof-ups, and he used to come back about every six months to clinic and come up to the unit to visit us, and everybody had given up hope on him, totally, because nobody knew what was wrong with him. He was so sick we couldn't figure out anything. He came out of his coma. All that time period he was in a complete coma from his metabolic deficiency.

Finally, Walker addresses the issue of resource allocation: who gets the ICU bed? Although the Lewandowski study indicates that adult DNR patients were commonly in ICU beds, the situation with pediatric patients may reflect the fewer ICU beds available:

Do you think that the ICUs usually work for children—that critical care is mainly geared for children who are salvageable?
Once there was a bed crunch where admissions needed to be governed a little bit more. In the older days when we didn't have quite the acuity level, there was not a strong line between that. A lot of patients who should have been hospice care or labeled "terminal," "do not resuscitate," on the floor were not, and they would have an arrest on the floor and end up—and anybody who arrested on any floor would end up in the intensive care unit, and once they came through the door, all support was given to them. We had Burkett's lymphoma, leukemia kids, all kinds of oncology and neurological—degenerative neurological diseases that used to come in. And then, once the acuity level rose, some big decisions needed to be made about that and then it did change and it was supposed to be only salvageable kids. So no terminal illnesses were supposed to be admitted to the intensive care unit at all, unless it could be

proven that it was an isolated incident that they wanted treated. Like, if it was during a chemotherapy induction they had a blood pressure dive, or something happened, and they would admit them until that problem was over and then they were to go back to their normal care. But that stayed a controversy always, and I'm sure it always will be. It's better now, I think, but about five years ago that was a big problem. And then when you'd get a newborn in with five to ten defects. You know, should they have been admitted? But see, that was different, because they weren't diagnosed until after they got there, and you found out what all the problems were.

Barbara Bauer describes a situation where the nurse was seen as accessible and approachable by family members when the physician was not able to make a decision about brain death:

What ethical decisions have you made or seen made in ICU by nurses?

I think probably the one that's closest to me right now is a patient that we knew had infarcted her brain stem and was moribund and the physicians refused to accept this. The family came to me asking for a decision and I said I would intervene with the physicians if that was their wish, and I tracked down the doctors and got everybody together without actually making the decision. It was hard on me because I knew this woman would not survive, but the physicians weren't willing to give up the ghost. We had a neurologist who said, "She'll be fine, she'll breathe on her own." We had to get a court order with this particular woman to have her taken off the ventilator, and she was dead within fifteen seconds—no spontaneous respirations and heartbeat.

How long had she been moribund?

About a week—but we very seldom are put in that sort of position, you know, a life and death position.

Bauer goes on to discuss the difficulties involved in nursing care of patients who do not do well after surgery. She describes the problems of patient selection:

The other ethical issue that we, as nurses, have nothing to do with is the pre-selection of patients. You know there are a lot of patients that we as nurses—and we've laughed with a few physicians about it—there's no way I would want my father, age 77, who's in perfectly good health, such as he is—I wouldn't want him going through mitral and aortic valve replacement right now. He might do well, but I'd have second thoughts about it, you know, if he could be treated medically. It just seems like so many of these patients, you know, when you start getting the 79- and 80-year-old patients with pre-existing, multiple health problems coming to you and just being sucked into the system. And then you end up with them as patients, and you have to turn to their families. For me that's as much a difficulty as anything else, turning to the families and saying, "Well, Mama just didn't wake up after her surgery." Or "She woke up, but she's not moving her right side. She's never going to be the same mother you knew or wife you knew or what have you. I'm sorry." That is difficult.

Bauer describes the difficulties of dealing, as a nurse, with the consequences either of decisions made by others, especially if the nurse perceives they were not in the patient's best interest, or of decisions that others just won't make:

Yeah. You know I had no choice over Mrs. Smith going to surgery. You know, I don't know whether she was railroaded into it by her family or it was a conscious decision on her part. But you see some of these patients who are like, my God, what ever made you think that your mother was going to do well in surgery? And I guess I have a tendency to relate it to my mother and my father. And sometimes you want to be angry with the family and you know you can't be and then you want to be sympathetic with the family and you just—you're very angry, and then you become angry at this party and usually it's, "How did Dr. So and So ever take Mrs. So and So to surgery knowing that she was blind in one eye, had bilateral mastectomies, and was a diabetic in renal failure, and he decided he was going to fix her heart and that was going to fix everything?" And you know, I'm not the only one who shares that. Sometimes when you see these patients, that's usually when you get the most discouraged. You see this little lady there and say, "My God, just send her home on her digitalis and Lasix." You know she's going to be in congestive failure. Maybe she'll have six months of better quality than we're going to send her home with. She may have a stroke and aphasia and be unable to speak or understand and six months later she'll probably be dead anyway. That's the hardest part for me and I think I probably share that with many nurses—I've talked with a couple of nurses that I work with, more than a couple, and that's probably the most frustrating thing.

Pat Dalton addresses issues of language and informed consent. Patients can't really know what the consequences of treatment may involve if things do not go well. Dalton describes the impact on the nursing staff of providing that care:

I don't think we inform people enough. And I don't think that our so-called "informed consent" is really informed. They don't realize what they're going to be put through. But we go round and round all the time. We've got one surgeon that does open hearts on some of these patients that are high risks. He did a case—it's been a couple of months ago, but it was on a—he was a 54-year-old man . . . had been turned down at the Cleveland Clinic and the Mayo Clinic five years ago because he was such a poor risk. He had such bad heart disease. And this particular surgeon decided he was going to do him. He ended up in surgery a long, long time. He had a hard time getting him off bypass, and they were going to put a left ventricular assist device in him and all this kind of stuff. They finally got him off. The surgeon was there waiting for the patient to roll around, and I asked him, "Why did you do it?" This particular doctor, he's only a couple of years older than me and I know he gets upset when his patients do badly and he gets real depressed when they die and it's a drain on him. But he said, "This man wanted it. He knew that if he didn't have it he was going to die and he wanted to take the chance." He said, "I had to do it." And this man did fine. Yet then we get another patient, the same surgeon did her. It was a young woman. She was about 40. But she looked about 30, I couldn't believe it. She was a real nice lady. She had no risk factors, but had a right ventricular AMI [acute myocardial infarction] all of a sudden. She wasn't a smoker and had no risk factors at all. She looked like a good risk for surgery. And he did her, and she died that night. So you never know, and I guess even though we say, "Why are we doing this to all these people?" If it's their choice, who are we to say, "No, we're not going to do it." But then again, these people have got to know what can happen to them. Physicians always say, I don't know how many times I've heard it, "Well, everything that's wrong with them can be reversed." Well, that's fine, but if somebody's in respiratory failure, is in cardiac failure, is in renal failure, or liver failure, and is comatose—sure, each one of them may be reversible, but don't tell me that you know that person's going to get up and walk out. You just don't see that. We had a trauma. A young girl. I know she was young, but had 40 units of blood in like a three-hour period. And you know right away that person's lungs are gone. They might as well forget that. Yet in the three-day period after that she must have gotten a hundred and more units of blood. And they tried to dialyze her and they did all that stuff. And she still died. They could have stopped days before and saved the family from any false hope that maybe she can get better, let alone from the expense people are being put through.

It's real frustrating when you see this. There's all this thing with informed consent with these open hearts. The physicians now are documenting in their progress notes, "The surgery was explained and the risk was explained for mortality, for bleeding, for stroke, was all written out for the patient with percentages." Nobody will ever convince me that these families and these patients realize that this risk for stroke could mean you're going to end up a vegetable for the rest of your life or on a ventilator for the rest of your life. They don't know what it means to be on a ventilator for the rest of your life. It's one thing if they tell you your risk of dying in surgery is 10 percent. Fine, if I'm going to die in surgery I'm going to die there, but they don't realize what it means to sit on that ventilator for the rest of your life. They don't realize what it means. They're told there's a one percent chance of infection. Big deal. People get infections all the time. They don't realize the sternum can get infected and it comes open and you can see their heart beating and we're putting dressings on top of the heart. They don't realize what that means, you know. And we keep doing it to these people. That's what is real frustrating to me. And we're seeing it more and more now too.

Karen Adler addresses the issue of "no code," meaning no care — who gets an ICU bed — and the issue of language:

I think that one of the major ethical dilemmas is an on-going situation and I am beginning to understand why physicians are hesitant to write a "no code" order, because a lot of nurses—once they see "no code" it also means no more care. That bothers me. To me you can have a "no code" that would mean that you were giving aggressive care up to the point that if their heart stops you are not going to resuscitate them. I have a hard time dealing with that, but the unit that I worked in before I came here, once a "no code" was written they were automatically discharged from the unit. The physician had no choice about it.

Do you think that nursing is in control of that? What makes that happen? If the nursing supervisor sees that you have a "no code" and that means no care then they may pull staff to another unit?

Exactly. If you have got three "no code" patients up here it should be fairly light. That doesn't really always mean "light." There are some "no codes" that you do back off on and that you do just drop down to every four-hour vital signs, but just because you write "no code" does not mean that the situation is going to happen. I have heard nurses when I have given them report for the next shift say, "He is a 'no code.' We are going to drop him down to four-hour vital signs," and nobody takes them to task for it so I guess it happens by default. Some physicians are really specific and say, "We are not going to resuscitate, but I still want every two-hour everythings."

Where should nursing be on that? Should nursing be determining that?

I think that it needs to be a joint effort to tell you the truth. I think that medicine and nursing need to sit down and decide, "Where are we going with this patient and what are we hoping for? Are we hoping that maybe he is going to pull through this situation and that he is partially salvageable, or are we saying that there is no hope at this point and we ought to let him go as quickly as possible?"

What about patients who are not salvageable, who keep getting all of this "stuff"? Do you have problems with that?

Yes, I have a problem with that. There are some physicians that you know that you will not get a "no code" out of them under any circumstances. It is just horrible. The family gets so upset when they finally realize what the code situations means, what you are doing with that patient at the very end.

What do you mean?

By coding. The best story that I have about that was I was taking care of a young leukemic one time and his father was a psychiatrist. For some reason it crossed my mind to ask him if he knew what it meant when we put him on a ventilator, that he was not going to be able to communicate with you, he will not be able to talk, and he said no, that he had no idea. I said we have to put a tube down him; that is the only way. It really threw them off for a few minutes. They did not know what they were agreeing to. How do you explain that to someone?

So providing information then is something that you do to help work out the difficulty. Do you see nurses doing that sort of thing independently?

Yes, I do. I see nurses doing that quite frequently.

Do physicians do it?

I am certain that they do but I have not seen that. I think that a lot of times the physician makes that decision independently without ever talking with the family. I have just had too many families walk in and say that if they had had any idea that this is what was going to happen to Mom I would never have gone through with this and I want it stopped. Once it is on, there is no way to stop it.

Most families and patients, you are saying, don't differentiate exactly what a code means?

Exactly. I think probably one of the hardest things is just dealing with the families and helping them work through their acceptance of what has happened to that point. This is important, particularly if they have had somebody who has gone through a successful code and is now on life support. The patient you are pretty much keeping comfortable with narcotics. That is one thing that we do with patients that are on ventilators is to keep them as comfortable as one can be in that situation. The families just have to sit and watch all of that, and I think that is one of the main problems, dealing with the families.

You said earlier that one of the most satisfying things about nursing in critical care was to make a difference. What kind of difference can you make in a situation like that?

A lot of times, one of the things that I say to families all the time is that you did the absolute best that you could under the circumstances. You made the decision that was best for everybody involved at that moment. Just giving them permission so that they don't have to feel so guilty about what has happened. I think that is where nurses do make a lot of difference in giving a lot of emotional support to families of terminally ill patients and then clarifying what all this means.

Terry James addresses the ethical issues that she has confronted:

I think one of the dilemmas that is difficult is when your personal philosophy conflicts with the philosophy of the patient and family and I think it's sometimes very difficult when the patient and families want one thing, but if it was you and you had your choice you'd want another.

Give me an example.

For patients who appear to be very terminal, appear to have very little hope and it is your assessment that they are terminal, and then the families in particular want anything and everything that can be done on and on and on and on and on and they will not give up.

How does that influence the nurse?

I think it makes her very anxious. I think that many times nurses really interpret those as cruelties to the patients, that the suffering is prolonged, and I think it really is a conflict of her own values and the values of the other parties.

The previous series of interviews support many of the findings of the Lewandowski study about the ambiguities of caring for DNR patients in the ICU setting. Appropriate medical and nursing care requirements of terminally ill or hopelessly ill patients in the ICU setting remain uncertain and debatable due to many factors. The Lewandowski study deals primarily with appropriate levels of care for patients already designated DNR. The interview data reveal many other aspects of the ethical dimension of caring for patients who are brain dead or hopelessly ill.

First, nurses discussed the pain, stresses, and frustrations of dealing continuously with patients who are brain dead or hopelessly ill, when the family or physician, because of legal entanglement or philosophy, persist in denial or indecision about designating a patient DNR. Because nurses are there so consistently, they must deal with the consequences of decisions made by others as well as the outcomes of decisions others will not make. Nurses experience a great deal of conflict, for several reasons, if they perceive that decisions are not in the patient's best interest. Nurses are present continuously and implement the specifics of care. Family members often approach the nurses, rather than the physicians, for rationale or explanations about care the physicians have not offered. Decisions made or not made by physicians or family — for example, decisions to withdraw treatment or to refuse to treat or to treat aggressively in persons in older age groups — may conflict with the nurses' value system, beliefs, or professional judgment.

Second, nurses described the difficulties associated with the meaning of language and communication in the critical care setting. Nurses were caught in a situation of crisis when physicians, because of fear of lawsuits, lied to family members about brain death in children or when physicians were unable to come to a decision about when to stop aggressive treatment, designate a patient DNR, and allow the patient to die with dignity. Nurses, especially nurse managers, were often effective in these situations in helping to establish policies to facilitate decision making about brain death or "no code" procedures. Nurses also facilitated or initiated discussion with physicians about stopping treatment.

Issues of language also present complex dilemmas for nurses in critical care settings. The language of "informed consent" is difficult, even for the most conscientious physician. Patients must be presented with a range of risks and benefits by the physician offering a particular treatment. As treatment options have become more complex and invasive, the consequences of long-term management of complications in patients who do not do well become awesome. Nurses described the conflicts inherent in caring for persons who, in hope of a good outcome, chose a procedure, but did not do well.

The conflicts in this scenario are major components of the realities of contemporary critical care practice for patients, families, physicians, and nurses.

Patients hope for positive outcomes, and this hope may influence recovery. Success and failure are not yet predictable. Patients do well who should not, and others die who seem to be excellent risks. Families and patients, in crisis, often may not "hear" the risks as they are explained. Physicians, with varying communicative skills, may deny the possibilities of failure so much that they cannot express them. And even if the risks are explained, language may be inadequate to express the reality. People cannot really know what it is like to live on a ventilator for the rest of one's life. Similarly, infections rarely can be interpreted as seeing one's open chest or abdomen.

The third outcome of these interview data deals with the conflicts and stresses associated with caring for DNR patients. "DNR" may be interpreted as "no care" by nurses, physicians, family, or nursing administration, although the DNR patient is often in ICU on a ventilator. Nurse staffing may often be reduced by management and actual levels of care may be reduced by nurses themselves, although the DNR patient's care requirements are, as Lewandowski notes, often equal to that of acutely ill patients. Nurses often experienced conflict over being caught between family members and physicians regarding degrees of aggressiveness in care, the absence of clear and honest communication, and implementing specifics of care they believed were causing pain or were not in the patient's best interest.

Beverly Quinn reflects on her experiences with dying patients in community hospitals and with the preconceptions about age relative to "no code" issues.

Tell me about your experiences with dying patients. Do you think that nurses do special things with dying patients?

Yes. A lot of times. I remember one patient, in particular, they had flown in from somewhere, and she did not have any family with her at all, and evidently she had a history of pulmonary hypertension, a lot of respiratory problems. I believe that she had some kind of degenerative muscular disease also. She passed out on the plane, and they brought her to the hospital and put her on the ventilator and all that. We had her increased all the way up to 100 percent oxygen, and you could just see it in her face that she knew that she was about to die, and she would just hold your hand. Especially in situations like that when there is no family or if the family had gone home. And, a lot of times they are not there in time before the patient dies. Being there with the patient and holding his hand and trying to make him comfortable. Nurses are there to do that. I know that there are some nurses who can't deal with things like that.

They don't want to deal with it, but I think that is part of nursing, helping the patient during those last minutes.

Why do you think that some nurses don't know how to deal with it?

I think that it is probably just them, their personal thing. I guess some people just can't deal with death even if it is someone that they do not know.

What about dying patients in in the ICU?

They need the same care and support as the patient in an acute situation that you know is about to die. If the patient knows that he is terminally ill and they have made him a "no code," I still think that he requires just as much time as the patient there in an acute situation. Maybe your focus of care would be different. You need to do a lot of psychological support rather than a lot of physical-type things for the patient. I think that you need to be there as a support system for the patient just as much.

What are the ethical issues that you have found yourself involved in the ICU?

Should the patient be made a "no code," even in cases where the family wants everything done for the patient? It might be a 99-year-old patient and the doctor comes in and puts in a Swan and does all of this. It is hard sometimes to know what would be the best thing. Should he just let the patient go? Should he should be doing everything for this 30-year-old but not this 99-year-old that he wants to put in a Swan and a pacemaker and all this stuff? Sometimes it is hard to decide what you think would be best or what should be done.

What about "no code" situations?

When I was at the community hospital last year, something that I felt I could not really understand, they had patients who were "no codes" and patients that were "chemical codes," and sometimes they would say "slow codes." That was real difficult for me. I felt that either you code a patient or you did not code a patient. For example, a patient that they made a "chemical code." I had never really heard of a "chemical code." If the patient went asystole [heart stopped] or the patient went into ventricular tachycardia [rapid, ineffective heartbeat] you would use the drugs, but you would not use any other kind of resuscitative measures. I could not understand that, especially if the patient was on the floor and wasn't on any kind of monitoring system. How could you make the patient a "slow code"?

How would you know their rhythm?

When I was a supervisor there, if the patient was a "chemical code," I told them they had to be on telemetry [cardiac monitoring]. That was a decision that I made, and I think that should be written into the policy. If they are going to be a "chemical code" on the floor, they should be monitored because you can't go in and say or guess that they should get this or that. That is one decision that I made that I thought was an ethical decision.

Norma Edwards, 32, has spent ten years in cardiology and in a coronary care unit in a teaching hospital since 1977. She speaks of the nurse's role in facilitating communication between physicians and families:

Frequently we get into situations of whether or not to make someone a "no code." The family requests that the doctor do it or vice versa.

How do nurses intervene?

I think by being pretty vocal to the physician and opinionated to the physician and supportive to family members.

How does communication happen in those situations?

Usually it is initiated by the nurses—it just depends. Sometimes it is a situation with the family initiating to the nurses because the doctors are unable to hear. I think that the doctors and the nurses are pretty open and honest with each other about it. Communication to the family is just supportive.

What is the most difficult part of those situations?

I think that the major stress and the hard part is before the decision is made. Once the decision is made and we know where we are going with it, it's not easy, but the real stress is over and you can be supportive or you can be aggressive because you know what the plan is. You don't have to wonder. You know what the plan of care is. I aggressively seek out communication between the doctor and the patients, family, and all this, but I pretty much support the doctors and patients. I have seen ethical decisions to be made by those methods.

What is it that you think that nurses do that is the most important to the patient?

I think that they coordinate the other services with the patient. I think that, if it weren't for the nurses explaining what is going on and why, there would be a lot more turmoil and misunderstanding between doctors and patients. I think that they buffer between the different services.

What is it that nurses do that is most important to physicians?

They don't know it, they are not aware of it, but the same thing goes for physicians. The nurses are buffering and being able and willing to answer questions, detect problems early in the patient that the physician only sees twice a day and can't anticipate to pick up those problems before they become acute. This is real important to communicate that. To look and search and shop for the right order, we do a lot of shopping.

Lee Usher speaks about the ethical dilemmas created by nurse staffing shortages and limited resources and by preempting death with dignity for patients who are terminally ill. Her strategy supports the observations made by Edwards that indecision and lack of communication create an ethical problem for patients, families, and nurses:

I think some of the ethical issues are keeping a patient alive when you know there's no hope. If you have enough nurses, then you can give the care to everybody. But if you have to spend your time taking care of somebody that you just know the returns are not going to be good at all, in fact you aren't going to have any returns, versus not doing for someone what you know you could do, then that is an ethical dilemma for nursing. I remember when I first heard about the Baby Doe regulation. I was in the university when that came out—and the first thing my mind flashed back to was the high-risk neonatal nursery at the city hospital and how I have seen nurses sit and cry because they just can't do everything and they knew they were working with this little preemie infant that didn't have a chance and they needed to be over there spending more time with the other one, and to me that is an ethical dilemma. It's a practice dilemma, but it has all kinds of ethics involved. That's what I'm talking about in giving the care to the person you know is not going to have a return. I'm not talking about just the regular care—keeping them clean and nourishing them and keeping them comfortable—the comfort measures. I believe that everybody has that right, and I also believe that you need to support them, that if they can come back, they will. But I'm talking about the absolute heroic measures that you know you can't do—I think some of the other ethical dilemmas that face nurses are whether you should resuscitate or not resuscitate. And you resuscitate unless the doctor has written the order, "do not resuscitate." Now if that's a team approach and that decision is made and everybody is respecting it and working with it, that's marvelous. But if you have to resuscitate someone that you know should not be resuscitated, and you know does not want to be resuscitated—

Or the family—

—or the family or whatever, but just because the doctor hasn't written the order, then I think that is a dilemma. It's a moral dilemma. It's an ethical dilemma.

A legal dilemma—

It's a legal one. It's a love dilemma, you know. You don't want to jump on someone's chest and put them through all of this if they could die with some dignity. I think that is a real big dilemma for nurses.

Nurses develop strategies for coping with these dilemmas themselves and also for helping patients and families survive the pain. Nurses need to have hope in patient situations, if not for patient survival or quality of life, at least for clear communication and decision making and death with dignity. Even when patient situations are hopeless and dehumanizing, nurses are there, continuously, with patients and their families. Nurses are there, caring for the patient, whatever the reality. Nurses are there in a personal way for dying patients when they were alone. They support family members to assist them in accepting the reality that they made the best decision possible at the time under the circumstances. Nurses implement policies that protect patients' rights when decisions about DNR status have not been made. Nurses facilitate communication between physicians and families and coordinate all hospital services dealing with the patients' care.

Finally, two experienced nurses discuss ways in which nurses cope with ethical dilemmas. First, Emily Vereen describes her role in working with dying patients, their families, and physicians:

I think that nurses help in identifying when the patient is tired, when the family or responsible person is tired and needs to discuss that issue. I think that the nurse observes when that patient starts to deteriorate to such a point, and she is probaby the catalyst for starting the discussions. I think that should be a nurse's major role. You start talking and preparing a patient, especially if there are children involved. Some husbands, some wives are not able to discuss it with children. Somebody has to prepare the children, and nurses are good at identifying strong role models in the family who can help them with that, or a minister, or friends. All those people are good role models for helping the family. I think nurses can help to identify those people and to help the patient himself. If you have established a good working relationship with the patient, death isn't taboo—I have been surprised as I listen and get open with a patient, how even patients who come to the hospital for basic simple procedures have many fears. Sometimes you forget that we expect that, unless you have the dreaded diagnosis of end-stage heart disease, or renal failure, or cancer, those people should be taking this routinely and not having fears. I find that patients who come in for simple procedures or for what we consider non-life-threatening reasons have an enormous amount of fear attached. I think that nurses can identify so much more than physicians can, because patients tell more things to nurses than physicians. They tell nurses things that they don't tell spouses, that they don't tell mothers and fathers. I probably know so many secrets, so therefore I think that we are a good catalyst for people to make some of those decisions. I have helped patients to finalize their wills, to tell people that they care about that they are dying, to make apologies to people that they felt that had wronged all of their lives. They want to make a final right, but still do not have the courage to say so. I have done so many things that don't have anything to do with nursing, but on the other hand it has to do with the spiritual health of that person. Nurses definitely have a big role in that, helping physicians even come to grip with the fact that it is time. I find that physicians get caught up in "I really wanted to save this person." Physicians have difficulty sometimes in understanding when it is time to stop, because especially in young patients they feel a frustration of not being able to do anything for a young person who is dying for whatever reason, whether it be from an injury or malignant disease, whatever the cause. If it is a young person, it is very hard for them to let go and give up and let that individual die. Sometimes you have to come to them and say, "It is just time that we start to talk about this just in case." Usually, once you pull their coat tails they realize that maybe they are being a little bit unreasonable and a little too optimistic and maybe a little too ego-bound on what their capabilities are going to be, so it is an important area.

Finally, Edith Hardeman describes her experiences with coping with ethical dilemmas in nursing practice:

What are the ethical dilemmas for you?

I think probably the biggest thing that we are dealing with right now is when to quit. I think that we have gotten to the point, remember this horrible song, I don't know when it came out, in the seventies, I think, maybe late sixties, but the words were, "It's good news week. Someone's dropped a bomb somewhere, contaminated the atmosphere and blackening the sky. It's good news week. Someone's found a way to give the rotting dead the will to live, go on and never die, have you heard the news?" Sometimes that song gets going on in my head. We're supporting every function in the body, but they are not living. They certainly are not living the kind of life they would want to live. I find that I had to look at it from the whole philosophical approach. When I was at the Catholic University of America, they could not make us take religion, but they could make us take philosophy. They made you take philosophy that was taught by a priest. We are faced with the situations where people are saying to us, "Don't let me die." You are sitting there with all this stuff around the room and thinking, "At the rate we are going we won't ever let you die. You will be here forever." Or the person who just can't be weaned off of the ventilator who says, "I am ready to die." There have been three patients in the last year, and I have been involved with all three of them, who wanted to die, who were ready to go. They talked about it with you, and they said, "Look, I am never going to get off of this machine. I am never going to get off of the ventilator. I am never going to live the kind of life I want to lead. I am ready to die. I want to be taken off of this machine. I don't want to live this way anymore." We had a man who said that to us. He was a minister. He said, "I want to die." It dragged out for three weeks of dual consults, dual psychiatric evaluations, dual this and dual that. Everybody kept saying, "This man, he wants to go. Can we tell him no?" It was very difficult because what we ended up doing was this. They decided that he would be given morphine, to be made comfortable. The ventilator would be gradually turned down and then turned off. It took a lot of morphine, and it took a lot of Valium and it took some Phenergan. It took a lot. It also took about five hours. I went into the room, and I said, "We are giving you your medicine now. Is there anything that you want? Do you want to see anybody?" He said, "No." He looked up at me and said, "Thank you" and said, "Good-bye." I walked out of the room, and I was dismissed, what can I do? We gave him the drugs and whatever he needed. I wasn't acutally pushing the drugs, but I was staying there saying, "Do you have a problem with this? If you do, I will do this. Don't take care of this patient if you can't handle this." You stay there until it is over. Just giving more morphine than you think you probably ought to, except that—It is very difficult these days because they can't live without the machines and they don't want to live with it. They are not crazy, what do you do? How far can you go in saying you will live, in spite of yourself? They are saying, "This isn't living."

The last two interviews reveal, in a very personal way, the qualities of the nursing care that can be given to dying patients. Nurses are there and are willing to be available to dying patients. They sense when patients are tired and ready to die. They also may support physicians as they work through their own grief in the process of letting someone die. Hardeman observes, "You stay there till it is over." Helping someone to die is painful, but almost a gift. The dehumanization of the artificial life support is far worse.

The ethical dilemmas experienced by nurses seem related to rapid changes in medical technology that often outpace structural and human adaptation and to the roles that nurses assume with patients, families, and physicians in critical care settings. Nurses are the single most persistent factor in the care of critical care patients. This presence involves nurses in the ambiguities of care of patients with multi-system failure and in care of patients where right to die, DNR, and quality of life are significant issues. Nurses are also involved in the types and levels of treatment that DNR may mean in patient care.

The ethical dilemmas created when extraordinary treatment was initiated or continued inappropriately and patients were not allowed to die with dignity caused much stress and conflict for the critical care nurses interviewed for this study. The major sources of stress seem related to the following factors. Nurses are at the bedside continuously and are carrying out the procedures that may be perceived by patients and by the nurses themselves as cruelty and torture. Indecision by others, especially family or physicians, may prolong this period of dehumanization. Physicians and nursing administrators may be more oriented toward "cure." Although care for DNR patients remains demanding and time-consuming, medical support in patient management and nurse staffing in units with DNR patients may actually be diminished. Especially in cases where decisions are not made, nurses may be the persons required to initiate resuscitative efforts on hopelessly ill patients if they die before DNR decisions are made.

The roles that the critical care nurses in this study assumed to cope with these ethical dilemmas were essentially the same roles that they assumed in other patient care situations. Significantly, as patient care becomes more complex, nurses continue to be involved in both independent and interdependent ways. Nurses reported involvement in initiating policy changes in hospitals related to brain death legislation. Other nurses described experiences of carrying out the actual care of patients, who, after court orders were obtained, were made comfortable and removed from life-support systems.

Nurses spoke of other roles that they used in caring for patients caught in these ethical dilemmas. These roles and behaviors include advocacy; management and coordination of the total patient care situation; communication with patient, family, physicians, and others, especially interpretation of the medical environment for the patient and family; shared intimacy with patients and an ability and willingness to use that for the patient's well-being; assessment of subtle changes in patient status and identification of trends; physical presence with patients who are dying, especially those who are dying alone; physical care and comfort measures; and support of patients, families, and physicians in the realities of painful decision making. Nurses voiced repeatedly in these interviews that their motivation for and major satisfaction with nursing rests in making a difference in the lives of patients in crises. That nurses report having been able to do this so persistently, in such diverse settings, despite rapid change, stresses, and a host of other inhibiting factors, seems to make this a pivotal issue for consideration as society deals with the problems of maintaining adequate nursing care.

5. Critical Care Nurses Speak

The purpose of this study has been to acquire and interpret, through the techniques and methods of oral history, interviews with critical care nurses. Nurses as individuals and nursing as a discipline are obscure in written histories. Nursing is often viewed in the shadow of the history of medicine, and even when the story of nursing is told, problems exist in finding appropriate primary source materials. While the details of nursing education and professional organization are well documented, the story of the development of actual clinical practice is almost non-existent. Further, written histories of nursing almost always demonstrate region, class, and sex bias; most written histories represent the activities of middle- and upper-class, northeastern white women. The development, since the 1960s, of clinical specialization has received even less attention by scholars.

The development of critical care nursing is tied to developments in medical specialization after World War II and the increasing use of highly complex technology in the hospital care of patients. The trend to locate very ill and dependent patients with highly skilled nurses began with the recovery room experience in the 1940s and 1950s. Improved techniques in cardiac surgery and developments in equipment for monitoring and manipulating cardiac status at the bedside accelerated this trend. The surgical and medical intensive care units (ICU) appeared in the 1950s and the coronary care units (CCU) in the 1960s. By the late 1960s, ICUs and CCUs were common in American hospitals of all types and sizes. Community hospitals would commonly have a large combined medical-surgical ICU and a separate CCU, while university teaching hospitals might have multiple ICUs representing medical and surgical specialties such as heart surgery, pulmonary, organ transplant, burn care, and the like. Patients in the 1990s might be admitted to an ICU for an acute illness like a heart attack; for short-term management after specialized surgery such as removal of a brain tumor; or for long-term management of complications of either, such as respiratory support on a ventilator after a postoperative stroke or pneumonia.

Political, economic, and social realities have changed the U.S. health care establishment and the populations requiring care. Americans are older and sicker at every age when they arrive for treatment at the largely "illness-oriented" and "crisis-oriented" medical system. Increasing numbers of individuals are denied access to medical treatment in the United States, and these factors have supported the call for reform of the health care system. The highly invasive medical and surgical interventions available in medical care require a complex technology, very specialized and skilled medical and nursing support, and multiple ancillary personnel and support structures. While these interventions result in effective treatment and improved longevity for many, the outcomes for persons who do not do well are severe. These individuals may spend their last days in impersonal environments, on life-support equipment, among strangers. Further, procedures and decision making regarding the use or discontinuance of extraordinary life support technologies are unclear and incremental, respectively.

These acute care and life-support scenarios occur daily in critical care units. Nursing is the persistent factor in the development and operation of the critical care unit. Specialization in nursing followed that of medicine. At the same time many technical support occupations emerged to manage the developments in medical technology. Nursing embraced the technology, acquired the skills, and assumed the task of teaching new nurses critical care content. The nurse, the patient, and the equipment "became" the critical care unit. Nursing incorporated these skills into traditional roles. While other groups concentrated on one system or focus — such as respiratory care or mobility — the nurse assumed total responsibility for round-the-clock care of the patient and all equipment that appeared at the bedside, although the ICUs might be distinguished by medical or surgical specialty.

The direct care role of the nurse has become very complex and sophisticated. The nurse maintains the equipment, generates vast amount of data, and makes decisions about patient care based on assessment of the data and the patient's total physical and emotional status. Frequently, the nurse initiates, modifies, or terminates treatment based on those assessments. Physicians and others depend on the nurse to call them to the patient's bedside when they are needed. In addition, the nurse "extends" the physiological or psychological functions of person's unable to care for themselves due to illness or injury. For example, the nurse will turn paralyzed patients and facilitate bowel, bladder, and skin integrity and will manage the airway and manipulate oxygenation in patients on respirators, who are unable to breathe for themselves.

The ICU environment also has become very complex. Illnesses that place patients in ICUs are crises, often sudden, painful, and debilitating in their impact on patient and family. The nurse becomes the primary figure and contact person for family members. The ICU environment and patient care have become increasingly risky as a result of the use of toxic or dangerous products such as plastics, chemicals, drugs, chemotherapeutic agents and radiation, and the introduction of highly contagious and incurable diseases such as hepatitis B, non-A non-B (C) hepatitis, and Acquired Immune Deficiency Syndrome. Infectious and toxic agents of particular concern to pregnant women and to men and women concerned with genetic damage to themselves such as cytomeglian virus (CMV), radiation, and toxic chemotherapeutics are increasingly present in hospitals.

The ICU environment, the high technological and emotional demands of patient care, and the organizational styles of management in some hospitals have been found to be very stressful, often contributing to burnout in nurses. The impact of this environment has received the attention of Spicer and Robinson (1990), who propose a conceptual model of the critical care work environment. A nursing shortage has been persistent in U.S. hospitals since soon after World War II, but has assumed crisis proportions in the 1990s. Ninety-seven percent of nurses are employed, and even though the actual number of nurses has shown a steady increase for the past twenty years, the increase has not kept pace with the demand. This shortage is thought to be due to an increasing demand for nurses and a diminishing supply (Georgia Nurses' Association, 1988). At the same time that increasing numbers of highly skilled nurses are needed, fewer women are attracted to nursing and nurses in the field are leaving for other careers. L. H. Aiken, in considering the future of hospital nursing, proposes new roles or career tracks in hospital nursing, designed to parallel the organization of medical care in hospitals. Aiken cautions that, although hospitals must be financially stable to survive, "Overidentification with the concerns of management and preoccupation with the day-to-day operation of the institution divert nurses' time, attention, and perhaps even loyalties away from patients and away from the clinical challenges and common interests they share with physicians" (Aiken, 1990: 7).

Altruism and caretaking have been consistent themes throughout the history of nursing. The economics of nursing as a predominantly female occupation, the current nursing shortage, and the value of caring ascribed by society and by nurses themselves are some of the issues related to the altruism of nursing that scholars have not sufficiently explored. The combination of altruism and competence peculiar to critical care nursing remains unexplored in a systematic way. As Vreeland and Ellis (1969) have noted, warmth and sympathy are expected from ICU nurses together with objectivity and assertiveness. This conflicting demand contributes to the stress experienced by nurses in ICU settings.

This study has examined the evolution of critical care nursing from the perspective of the practicing nurse, through the use of oral history methods. It has attempted to answer several research questions. Five conclusions can be drawn from the interview data.

The nurse became the most persistent treatment figure in the critical care unit because of skill, competence in judgment, and round-the-clock presence.

The growth in technology, medical specialization, and knowledge focused the need to place the nurse with the patient in the critical care unit. The need to locate the nurse with the patient seems to be the guiding force behind this planning, rather than the need to manage the equipment. In fact, the early units in the 1950s opened without special monitoring equipment. The nurse was the monitor, and the private duty model seemed the appropriate one to illustrate this nurse-patient relationship. As technology changed continuously and very rapidly, the nurse added the new skills to the traditional caretaking roles that had been the domain of nursing. The nurse became the critical care unit. Vast amounts of data were generated, and again the nurse incorporated additional skills into the scope of practice. In fact, nurses had always made clinical judgments about patient care. But critical care increased the pace and the complexity of these judgments and subsequent acts.

Nurses perceived technology with ambivalence, appreciating the successful outcomes for patients but experiencing great conflict with its use. Technology was expensive and time-consuming and generated a great deal of data that often was not used appropriately. Medicine and nursing at times became overreliant on technology at the expense of the manual physical assessment skills of palpitation, auscultation, observation, and percussion. Roles became unclear, and questions became increasingly common about the appropriate uses of technology. The existence of technology, rather than individual patient need, often seemed to dictate its use. Nurses expressed frustration in those situations since the technologies were often invasive and painful for patients, and often the nurse was the person implementing the treatments. Technology compressed the time available to teach patients in even a minimal way about their illness. As technology became more pervasive, the human dimension of care seemed compressed and compromised.

The technology at the bedside — monitors, drug titrations, drains, infusions, everything attached to the patient — became the on-going responsibility of the nurse. The caring, skill, and continuous presence of the nurse were accompanied by a new aggressiveness.

The commitment of critical care nurses to patients and to nursing practice is passionate and personal. They believe that they make a difference to patients through competence, caring, coordination and management of the clinical environment, and advocacy.

The critical care nurses in this study expressed great commitment about self, nursing, and caretaking. Many described nursing as a vocation. Nurses believed that they made a difference in the lives of others in crisis through competence in the care delivered, management of the patient's clinical situation, and the relationship they established with patients and their families. Even nurses who were neutral about expressing a vocational commitment were heavily invested in patients, nursing, or the clinical situation. None of the nurses interviewed were indifferent, negative, or impersonal about patient care or nursing.

Nurses valued their patient contact even as the skill level increased. The nurse-patient interaction was the greatest source of motivation and satisfaction that nurses expressed. Hence, those same situations were frustrating when patients were caught in crises of indecision about the uses of technology, especially extraordinary treatment. Since nurses were constantly present with patients, patients and often their families confided secrets to nurses, and frequently the nurse would serve as mediator between patients and their physicians or their own family members. Nurses felt that they were a humanizing link for patients and families in the impersonal hospital environment. For example, the terms "instant intimacy," "taking care of patients," and "making a difference" were expressions used often to describe the kinds of communication, advocacy, and physical and emotional bond nurses experienced with patients. This was accomplished through teaching, interpreting the medical or hospital system, manipulating details of the environment to meet a goal, and performing multiple tasks simultaneously to "make the hospital system work for patients."

Performing many tasks at one time involved providing "hands-on" physical care, communicating with and coordinating many individuals and groups, and managing physiological imbalances in unstable patients. Nurses recognize subtle changes and patterns, and intervene before a crisis event occurs. Physicians are dependent on nurses for this function. Most often, the physician would not be aware of a patient problem unless alerted by a nurse. Nurses report special satisfactions and skill in caring for dying patients and for patients in pain. Nurses use touch, relaxation, and creative presence in these situations.

The satisfactions of intimacy with patients and the challenges of clinical care occur at a cost. Nurses indicated that many stresses exist in these environments. These stresses include: feeling responsible and in fact being expected to meet the totality of a person's needs when the nurse has limited authority for autonomous decision making; the care itself (for example, being constantly involved with dying patients); the constraints of the job (for example, lack of administrative support, inflexible hours, heavy demands, perceived low self-esteem, and inadequate staffing patterns in the ICUs); and the rapidly changing and complex technology, especially if indecision regarding its use results in prolonged patient suffering.

These increased levels of role functioning with patients, physicians, and others resulted in increased status and self-esteem for some nurses. Others expressed almost a schizophrenic ambivalence about nursing, hospitals, and medicine because of stress and the lack of clarity in their roles.

The ethical dimensions of critical care nursing, especially those that deal with death with dignity, are sources of conflict and stress for the nurses interviewed.

Nurses expressed great satisfaction when patients were allowed to die with some element of humanity and dignity, if death was inevitable. As painful as dying could be, artificial life support was worse, especially for nurses, because they provide the care that they may perceive as "torture" and "dehumanizing." Nurses felt so personally involved with patients that participation in such care was seen as a violation of patient wishes and a betrayal of trust. Conflicts in decision making among patients, families, and physicians were the major sources of stress in these situations. Nurses perceived that they often facilitated decision making and communication at these difficult times. They often recognized when patients were tired and helped communicate this to families or physicians. They also reported that they provided support to physicians when "it was time to quit." The dilemmas seem to emerge from the technological capacity to extend life. One nurse said, "The ability to do has outstripped the ability to decide when doing is appropriate."

The issues involved with "do not resuscitate" (DNR) were the most frequently cited dilemmas related to death with dignity. The stresses nurses experienced before DNR decisions were made resulted from the uncertainties about intervention. The nurse would be the person to initiate life support on a person for whom she perceived no hope of return to quality of life, if DNR decisions were not made before death. After the DNR decision was made, the stresses related to the ambiguities about appropriate levels of medical and nursing care. On the one hand, DNR care might be interpreted as all intervention except resuscitation. Often nurse staffing was reduced in ICUs if DNR patients were present. Some nurses reported that nurses themselves interpreted DNR to mean little or no nursing care.

This issue of appropriate levels of care portrays an underlying theme that has been persistent in the history of ICUs — who needs ICU care? Critical care has at times been interpreted as justified for those individuals who will recover to some quality of life. From this perspective, terminally ill patients do not require a critical care bed. These attitudes and values have been variable and influenced by the resources available — such as the number of ICU beds available or the level of financial reimbursement for services. Rapid increases in technology, the increased availability of ICU beds, and the highly invasive procedures performed in the 1990s have created a situation where many ICU beds are filled with patients suffering from the end-stage consequences of disease and/or treatment. These realities exist along with the differing views of who deserves ICU care. These issues have not been addressed, except in an economic sense. Hospitalization, treatment, and ICU care are generally available for those who can pay.

The incongruities involved in issues related to language, informed consent, and the realities of care of patients dying from the consequences of disease or failed treatment represented other ethical dilemmas for critical care nurses. Hope versus risk were very real, and language was inadequate to express the realities of "living the rest of your life on a ventilator" or "seeing your heart beating in your open, infected chest cavity." Nurses experienced these conflicts because of their commitment to patients and because they were there so constantly providing the care.

Nurses described the realities of caring for patients who, at their request, were removed from life-support equipment and allowed to die peacefully. In these situations, nurses were involved in facilitating decision making and legal processes and providing the drugs and emotional and physical support at the time of death. One nurse said, "You stay till it's over."

This persistence in caring and remaining at the bedside does have limits. Nurses reported a high degree of stress and burnout in ICU settings. The nurses interviewed represent nurses still active in nursing practice. Very little was found in the literature or heard in the interviews about successful measures to reduce nurse burnout. The issue is complex and likely related to the status and self-perception of women, the status and realities of nursing in hospitals, and the value of caring.

Nurses feel ambivalence and conflict about the necessary and difficult relationship between nursing and both medicine and the hospital as an organization.

As care became complex, nurses and physicians in critical care settings worked persistently and closely together. Both groups had specialized skills and communicated in complex ways. Ambiguities often existed in roles, relationships, male-female interaction, and distinctions of power and influence. Critical care nurses and physicians shared expertise and knowledge in various medical and surgical specialties that excluded other nurses and physicians. Nurses assumed many roles that had been within the traditional domain of medicine — physical assessment, determining drug dosage and titration based on physiological criteria, initiating or withdrawing invasive lines or tubes. This close association resulted in expert care for patients with particular problems, for example renal failure or heart transplant.

However, the priorities, values, and status of the two groups are often at variance. The physician retains the power of ultimate, formal decision making with regard to patient care. Nurses and some physicians (for example, specialists in anesthesia, radiology, and pulmonary medicine) are hospital employees and, along with consulting physicians, physical therapists and nurses are in a position to recommend or use formal and informal methods to influence care.

Nurses described several examples of frustration in dealing with physicians. These included indecision about designating a patient DNR; being deceptive with patients, families, or nurses; refusing to come and see critically ill patients when called by a nurse; and continuing painful treatment on patients against their wills, when death is inevitable, either because of research goals or physician denial. Nurses also reported instances of excellent rapport with physicians where they felt mutual respect for skill and support in coping with the shared losses in critical care. The relationship between nursing and medicine deserves further study relative to the changing status of medicine in U.S. society, the crisis of hospital care related to the nursing shortage, the support systems available to both medicine and nursing, and the changes in health care brought about by the increased focus on prevention and health promotion, a more informed consumer and managed care and prospective payment systems.

The conflicts in nursing practice related to the nurse as hospital employee represent an area that has received little attention by scholars. The personal commitment and nursing practice philosophy of the individual critical care nurse are directly influenced by how effectively a particular hospital is managed. Nurses described the stress and frustrations when nurse staffing was inadequate to provide minimally safe care to patients, when in fact hospitals could close beds to maintain adequate nurse-patient ratios or increase nurse-staff ratios. When these staffing patterns became rather frequent events, nurses exercised the only control they had. They left that hospital for another job or they left nursing for another career. Staffing patterns, more than any other, were described as the one final stressor that, added to the many others, made nurses consider leaving the setting or the occupation.

Nurses consistently expressed that "making a difference to patients" was their primary motivation for nursing. These same values were expressed by the nurses currently in administrative positions in hospitals. Yet practicing nurses experienced impotence and felt that they were treated with indifference by administrators. Nurses felt that they were valued less as individuals and more as anonymous pawns. "A nurse is a nurse is a nurse. I'm not valued as an individual or as a person of value." It is important to remember that the nurses voicing these feelings are the ones still in the settings providing the care. Nursing and hospital administrators would do well to examine the conflict between professional nursing practice and employment in the bureaucratic organization of the hospital. The private duty model, where patients and nurses contracted for service, exists in nursing history as a focus for study. Certainly, patients require adequate nursing care in hospitals, and that care must be provided efficiently. This issue may be one component of the problem with the U.S. medical care system.

Voices of critical care nurses reflect the values of the individual and the culture at any point in time.

The interviews with critical care nurses reveal a number of instances where issues related to race were apparent. These examples reflect attitudes and values of individuals, educational institutions, and hospitals at particular points in time in particular places. These observations should be taken in context, since the sample of nurses was predominantly white and female. Black women and one (white) man were included, but there was no representation from Asian, Hispanic, or other minorities or members of non-Christian religious groups. Many, but not all, of the examples of racial prejudice toward Blacks occurred in the South. A Black nurse reflected that Black patients and their families seemed to rely heavily on her in military hospitals, because of the comfort in racial affiliation. A young Black nurse reported that although she loves nursing she would encourage young Black females to pursue careers in medicine, law, or business. She reflected that, while her family saw nursing as upwardly mobile for a Black woman in 1979, she saw the economic and status advantages of the traditional male-dominated professions, now open to women, as upwardly mobile in 1987.

Two examples of the philosophy of educational institutions were provided. One fifty-eight-year-old Black nurse described her experiences as a nursing student in an urban, southern, segregated, hospital nursing school. She has remained a continuous employee of the hospital. She experienced integration and is now a nurse manager. Her story is a case study of the human experience of social change and a reflection of a contemporary urban hospital. A second nurse, thirty-five, described the dehumanizing experience of being required as a Caucasian baccalaureate nursing student in a white, private university to go to an urban outpatient clinic and "interview" to learn therapeutic, interpersonal skills. She described her resentment at being required to "use" patients and give nothing back to them that would benefit their care and her empathy for patients who felt compelled to be compliant and to participate.

Several examples of racial prejudice toward Blacks (and Jews) and the ways in which prejudice influenced the ranges of medical options offered and the quality of care provided were discussed. Two nurses described care provided in the South to siblings in crisis with sickle cell anemia. Both described indifferent medical care and spoke of nursing care that consistently underestimated pain. These nurses learned about comfort measures caring for these siblings at home, and both nurses reported that these experiences were a motivation for nursing as a career. Oral history methods seem useful in revealing the depth in these debilitating experiences.

A Black nurse described the cultural tradition in the Black community to reject the offer of "do not resuscitate" designation for patients who have no hope of recovery. She attributed this reluctance to mistrust of the white medical system and the fear that whites will not do all that they can to save Blacks. She also noted the characteristic faith in God in the Black community: "Man does all that he can and God will take care."

A white nurse reported that in hospitals in the north and south she had witnessed that fewer aggressive medical options had been offered to patients who were poor and Black. She felt that the philosophy of the attending physician and the degree of aggressiveness of family members were the primary determinants.

Finally, a white nurse reported that in two hospitals in the segregated South in the early 1960s she saw old surgical instruments labeled "colored" for use with Blacks. She opened a coronary care unit in a segregated hospital in South Alabama where Black hospital floors were not staffed with registered nurses but with aides, and Black patients were not admitted to the CCU even if all beds were empty. "Blacks didn't have heart attacks in Alabama," she said. She described an event in the emergency room where a white physician said "stop the code" on a black man who was responding to resuscitative efforts. She said, "They just didn't treat Black people. They let them die." These observations are valuable in pursuing the social and cultural history of a region and the personal story of nursing and health care.

A final interview was conducted with Jamie Marsh, a thirty-nine-year-old critical care nurse who discusses her experiences as a critical care nurse and describes her care of a family waiting for a heart transplant. The interview reveals, in a very personal and powerful way, the practice themes and dilemmas that have been discussed in this book. She begins with her early experiences as a nurse.

I was just thinking, I was a new graduate, had worked as a nursing assistant on a med surg floor. I wanted to work in ICU. I knew I never wanted to work on a floor even at that young age. And I was upset with the folks at the hospital where I was working, because they wouldn't let me go straight out of nursing school into the ICU. Well, in retrospect, I realize what a smart decision that was on their part. I went to work at another hospital, in an ICU there. They said that I would be trained, that I wouldn't be put in there all by myself. Well, I wasn't by myself. I was with a nurse who had never worked at all, not even as a nursing assistant. So I was in charge on the night shift, twelve-hour nights. We did open heart surgery at that hospital. They started off by doing heart surgery in the OR [operating room] on dogs and we would go down there and watch them; this was in '73. And we thought we were just really uptown. There was a respiratory therapist on days and one on evenings and nobody on nights. So, when we started doing open heart surgery, fortunately, we only had one patient at a time, respiratory therapy would come in there one last time before they left at eleven o'clock and check on the ventilator, and just told us not to touch anything until morning. And we did probably, in the year I was there, about ten. We probably did ten patients.

Did they live?

And they all lived. Now, it was purely by the grace of God, I'm certain. Maybe they were just incredibly healthy specimens to start with and—scary. And I had no idea how dangerous it was. I thought, "We're on the cutting edge of medicine here."

From dogs to this.

That's right. At least they didn't have fleas.

What was appealing about ICU? Why did you want to be in ICU?

I had floated in there a couple of times while I was working on the floor. It was my last year of nursing school. So I was in a nursing assistant/graduate nurse role. So what it meant was, you took on the nursing assistant's and the nurse's role at the same time. So you just did twice as much work. And we gave medicines. It was kind of scary in retrospect what all we did. We were team leaders, and this was without an instructor there. This was just, "Okay. Here you are and here's your team." And I remember I was 19 years old. I was a baby, and having some of these grouchy old LPNs who'd been in nursing forever—been out of school twenty to thirty years, and me trying to tell them how to do their work. That was eye-opening.

Most of your experience has been in ER [emergency room] and ICU?

The critical care areas. I think, because of the overwhelming nature of the floors, I could never get myself organized enough to handle—and at the time, that's been almost twenty years ago, you had twenty patients. There was a team leader, and maybe a medicine nurse, and a nursing assistant, and you had twenty patients. And I couldn't stand not knowing what was going on with all twenty of them. And it—I'm not really a perfectionist, but I do want to at least recognize my patients as mine and have them remember me as their nurse instead of—so many nights it was, you run there, "Hi, I'm Jamie, your nurse, you won't see me again," and I didn't like that.

Holler if you're really sick.

Yeah. "I hope your wife knows what she's doing."

So your work as a nurse has been pretty much in ICUs, and you've worked in a number of hospitals. Think about the organization of the hospitals or the units that you've worked in. What kinds of structures and processes enhanced care and inhibited it?

I think staffing is the biggest plus you can have. You've got to have good auxiliary staff. And that's one thing, I think, that appeals to me about my current hospital, and the reason I stay—I've been there the past ten years, and that's why I stayed, because they've got auxiliary staff, you've got transportation, you have a tube system. That tube system has saved me more time over the years, just being able to send slips where they need to go. But you have a transportation department that—for the most part, they really do know how to transport patients. We have patients with a lot of lines and tubes, and by and large I've seen that they're very careful and they know what they're doing, and that's important. But just having adequate staffing—money is important, sure, I won't kid you there. And here—I think I'm making more there than I could anywhere else right now because of the levels program. There again, it provides a lot of incentive. But I think adequate staffing to me makes or breaks a situation. When I was in the float pool, I got pulled to a floor that was a—it was a pilot program, it was an "all-professional floor." So they had no clerk and no assistants. And I was pulled over there, and I had three fresh post-ops and two coming back from surgery on an evening shift. I was pulling my hair out. I was ready to quit nursing because I had all these fresh post-ops that I wanted to check on, and being an ICU nurse you get a little more fastidious about what you want—what you think's important. I wanted to make sure that they got their care. And then here I come with two fresh post-ops, trying to get a couple of them up and down to the bedside commode, walking them up and down the hall, trying to take off orders, and I thought, what is so damn professional about this, you're running yourself to death and your patients are getting lousy care and you're ready to pull your hair out, and you're popping Maalox pills running down the hall. I said, "No, this is not professional." Professional is being able to orchestrate the care and be involved in it, but you don't have to do every single thing that patient needs. I think that they suffered in the long run. I know I did, and vowed never to go back to that floor.

Do you feel like most of what you do in your present situation is nursing care? Are you caught up in a lot of non-nursing stuff?

No. I think in our unit it's mostly nursing care. We have an excellent auxiliary staff. We have a clerk who knows what she's doing and she's there to do it, and we have excellent nursing assistants. Now, part of the reason I think our unit runs well is because of our nursing assistants. We have one who is in nursing school. He'll be leaving in a few months off to the grand world of nursing. And another one is majoring in physics, wants to be a medical engineer, whatever, one of those pump tech-type people, so we've got people that are motivated. But I have worked with some bad nursing assistants that would just as soon not have. But I think most of what we do is nursing care. We do a lot of teaching, a lot of interaction with the family, and our patients stay a long time.

What things interfere with your doing nursing care?

The things that seem to interfere with doing nursing care are when we are short-staffed or if our assistant calls in and we don't get one and you're bogged down doing all the mundane tasks. Being a medical ICU, we have patients, generally they are there a long time, a lot of them can't do anything for themselves, can't feed themselves, if they're even able to eat, maybe they're incontinent and they need a lot of just maintenance care, ventilator care, skin care. And you can't do that if you're not staffed. And we do a lot of teaching.

Tell me about George and Alice.

We have—there again, in our unit we have cardiomyopathies who are there a long time. We had one man that was with us for nine months before he finally got a heart transplant, and he's doing well. He brings us goodies, and he came back last summer and brought us a bushel of peaches. So, when we have our cardiomyopathies waiting on transplants, we assume that they are going to get a heart. We have not, in our unit, in the past six or eight months had a successful—a long-term patient that was successful at getting a heart. So George and Alice came to our unit last year. They're both in their forties, late forties, good folks, good sense of humor, really up-type people. They had one son who was really supportive, really supportive family, and we just expected that he was going to get a heart. He had a viral cardiomyopathy. He'd been a healthy—was a computer programmer. She was a medical assistant in a doctor's office. And we just expected that he was going to get a heart. We were all really close to him. He was ambulatory. He had his Dobutamine [to strengthen the heart muscle] and Heparin drips [to prevent blood clots]. But he was ambulatory. We went down for Easter services about this time last year, went down. He walked and had his little pumps on the pole. We walked down there, had Easter services, everybody—and then we walked to the front of the hospital, looked at the flowers. He wanted to go back down to the auditorium, make sure everybody was gone, and he started playing the piano. We never knew this about him, that he had had a love for the piano. Alice told us afterwards, when we discovered this flare, that he had a grand piano at home, and that was what he did to relax. And he played for an hour. There was a Baptist hymnal down there and he played just beautifully for an hour. I called back to the unit and told them that we'd be there, if they needed me to give me a page. So, after that, we got him—when we got back to the unit, we borrowed from rehab one of those big keyboards, and then his family brought in a keyboard, and he would sit in his room and play the piano. It was kind of a nice, uplifting corner of the unit. We had moved him to our biggest room with a view. He would take himself off the monitor with our permission and walk out to the little anteroom outside his room. His grandchildren would come up there and they visited. They had birthday parties up there for the families, and he would just—he was ambulatory, more or less self-care. We would take him out—if there was an empty room on the floor, we would walk him down there and he would take a shower. We had him off the monitor, we'd tape up his pic-line—after the first couple of months with us, he didn't have a Swan anymore. They would put a Swan in for a couple of days just to get the numbers to make sure he was all tuned up. But his numbers never changed, his medicine never changed, he was so stable. So we just assumed it'd be like the other guy we had; he'd be there for six, seven, eight months. The holidays kind of came and went, though. The Christmas holidays came, and we thought, "Okay. There's going to be some drunk out there New Year's Eve and he's going to get a heart." It never came. Spring came—that was a kind of standing joke, "Well, it's the weekend. All the good ole boys will be coming back from the lake with their beer and their pickup trucks and somebody's bound to smash into somebody and give you a heart," and it just never came. We would—we'd bring the kids up there; anybody that had come up to get their paycheck or whatever would bring the kids in and it was a family thing. He called my son one day from the hospital room, we'd been talking about some accomplishment he'd had at school, and he called and they chatted, they talked about baseball. He was involved in our lives and we were involved in his. And his wife, Alice, just made us all feel at home. She had set up camp outside the room, had the cot and all her little goodies, had a little cooler out there, and had her own little corner that was sort of a dresser-type thing. We just all felt real comfortable. For the most part, the same nurses took care of him all the time. But we felt like he was our baby; although you couldn't really say he was a baby because he was a very independent man. He took care of his business and we took care of ours, and on the off moments, if we just wanted to escape from the hectic pace of the unit, we'd just go in there, we'd exchange jokes. He was full of jokes, and we'd bring them to him, and he'd give them right back to us. He had a lot of visitors. It was a very normal-type of life style. He really felt at home, he and Alice both. And since he died, his wife and I have corresponded on numerous occasions.

So what needs did he have?

Physical needs?

What did nursing do that made a difference for him in terms of his needs—you mentioned maintaining normalcy was one thing.

That's what I was going to say. I think he needed to be in control as much as possible. And we were able—because he was stable—because he was so stable for so long, we were able to provide that control. He—part of it was taking himself off the monitor, and he'd let us know. He'd beep the button and just say he's going to go sit out in the waiting room for a while. And that was cool; he was stable. It wouldn't have worked for a lot of patients, but we—his wife was with him. He had a pacemaker and an AICD; we figured that—at worst, you know, his AICD would kick in and shock him while we were running out there. But he wasn't in imminent danger of death. But the main reason he was with us was just because he couldn't get off his drips and he needed to stay there until he got a heart. I think his wife being there all the time and being as supportive as she was, his family coming in, and then him being able to maintain the control over his environment to a certain degree. Now, we knocked before we went in that room. If the door was open, it was an invitation, anybody could come in, but if the door was closed, you needed to knock, because that was his domain. He and his wife might be smooching in the corner somewhere, and we respected that. In fact, he told a funny story. He was getting his shower one morning—not a shower, but getting—bathing at the sink right behind the curtain, Dr. Roberts just sort of barged in, he didn't know our routine. Well, George and Alice were, I forgot how he put it, "getting some lovin'," something to that effect, behind that curtain, and he was off the monitor, and Dr. Roberts walked in and just didn't say anything, they didn't know he was there, and he just pulled the curtain open. Well, Dr. Roberts, bless his heart, I never saw a U-turn so fast; so George laughed about that for a long time, they both did. So it was a pretty normal situation. Sometimes she would curl up in the bed with him. There was never any sex, but there was a lot of intimacy. So he was able to maintain that control. And even before he went in the hospital—we didn't know this at the time when he came in—but he had made sure that everything was taken care of at home. He had had a security system put in, he had extra lights outside, they had worked—ever since he was diagnosed with his cardiomyopathy, they had worked extra hard to pay off the house; and they paid the house off. He says that he never really expected to get a heart, but if he did he was glad for it. But it didn't make him a pessimist. I think he was much more of a realist. He had written letters to his wife in case of his death where all the important papers were, what the bills were. He had planned his funeral, what he wanted played, what kind of service he wanted, who he wanted to be pallbearers, where he wanted to be buried. He had made all those plans. And talking about it, it sounds like he was a real control-oriented person. But I didn't get that impression just knowing him. He was just a very pragmatic person who took care of what he could and left the rest to fate, God, nurses, whatever. But they were very special folks, and

of the external environment, not the patient's environment, but what goes on on the outside to allow that patient to get some rest. I can't tell you how many times over the years we've either stopped a lab person, or respiratory, or even a doctor from barging in and disrupting what you've carefully orchestrated to try to maintain some rest.

You told me that, when you were getting the new monitors and also the new pumps that beeped all the time that everybody hated, that George learned how to use them and learned all about them.

He'd tell you how to use it. Do you know what he said to me? I had forgotten this until right this minute, he said, "I'm beginning to think that my name is 'oh, shit.'" That's what he said. He said, "First you have to cuss at it." Then he said, "This is the third time a nurse has come in here and said, 'oh shit.'" Yeah. Well, it is a small pump and that's the only reason we left it on him, even with all of the alarming, because he was so ambulatory.

What is it that nurses did that was most important to him? Do you have a sense of that?

I think just being his friend, being a confidant. He had—some nurses didn't care for him, didn't care for his personality, so those of us that did always took him as our patient. Sometimes I think he got to be the—he was so stable we would almost pair him—if we had to, pair him with somebody who was really busy. So sometimes he got neglected. But I don't think he really minded that. We would go in there a lot of times just to blow off steam. You'd go in there after something bad had happened or whatever and you could just talk to him about it. So I think he met our needs as much as we met his. But he would—he had several of us, four or five that I can think of, that were really confidants, and he would tell us what he wouldn't tell the doctor or what he wouldn't tell the psychiatrist for sure, things that he knew would never be passed along, some of his feelings. A couple of times—and he told me, he said, "I know that this won't go any further, because if this were told a psychiatrist it would be twisted in such a way and put on the chart that I'd look like a psychopath." So he would—I really think in terms of caring for him, the physical needs were important. Obviously, we had to make sure that the drips were right and that sort of thing, but for most of his time there and really excluding the last week of his life, he wasn't particularly sick. He was tuned up and stable. So his needs were more emotional and, I guess, friendship-type-related needs.

Was that what was important to Alice?

Yes. Yes. She enjoyed the camaraderie. She felt comfortable with us. We talked a lot, not just the two of them and myself, but the four or five nurses that really got close to him on a much more personal level. Some people, like I said, just didn't care for his personality or didn't understand that everything—he kidded a lot, and they just didn't like it or maybe they couldn't relinquish control. I think the nurses that really did get close to him were some of the older nurses who maybe have gotten over that need for control.

How do physicians react to long-term management of care?

I think part of the problem—now, this is strictly a biased comment and it's not based on any medical evidence. He had been rock stable until we—they changed fellows. There was a changeover and this new fellow came in and decided that he wanted to change the regimen. He wanted to get him off his Captopril and put him on Vasotec. He wanted to wean him off the Dobutamine and put him on something else. And when they started messing around with his drugs, he started a gradual decline. And we put—we finally got him back on his other regimen, the previous one, and he was better. But he just never got back to that level where he'd been before. And I really blame this person. There again, I'm not looking at it very objectively because I liked George and Alice so much as people that I wanted them to get a heart and live happily ever after, almost as much as he did, I think. And when they started messing around with his fluids and with his medicines, he just started a downhill decline. And the attending physician is a really nice guy and I like him a lot, but he's not likely to rock the boat. So the fellows seem to be doing most of the management of the care, the fellows and the nurses. The nurses had a lot of input with what worked and what didn't. The docs started screwing around with the schedule. I think that was his demise. And they wouldn't listen to us. I went round and round with this guy one morning and trying to pin him down about some things and make him comply to the way that I wanted it done, and he just got really defensive and just walked out of the room, just left, left the unit, never came back, never answered my questions. We just never got this resolved.

The fellow?

The fellow. And he said, "I'm doing the best I can," and left. Of course, we didn't think that was good enough. I had a doctor tell me once, he said, "I don't know why they call it doctor's orders. They should just call it doctor's suggestions because y'all are going to do what you want to anyway."

What is it that nurses do that's unique that other people don't?

Oh, I think the most unique thing about nursing is they can take—I look at nursing like there's a patient in the—it's almost like the spokes on a wheel—there's a patient in the middle and the nurse surrounds herself around that patient and then all the other spokes of the wheel are the doctors, the pharmacist, dietary, central supply, everybody else that comes in contact with that patient. And that nurse has to insulate the patient from all those other spokes and act as a liaison and act as a—sort of a conduit to make sure that everybody does their job for the benefit of that patient.

Is that primarily in ICU or is that why working on the floor is so frustrating, or being busy, because you can't do that?

I think so. Yeah. That's probably why. I hadn't really thought about it in those terms. Because I definitely feel like the one who insulates that patient, who is truly the patient advocate and probably the only patient advocate, the only person who can look after—to look at all the aspects of care, not just whether or not he gets the right medicines or whether or not his food is right or whether that X-ray gets done. The nurse is the one that coordinates it all and I think is such an integral center of that wheel.

Is that how you would define nursing?

Yeah, I think so. I think so. We do for the patient what he can't do until he can do it. That sounds like Orem's self-care model, but—

Well, it sounds like Virginia Henderson to me.

Okay. Well, I haven't learned about Virginia yet. But I don't think that we can look at the patient in the terms of specific deficits. I think you have to look at the whole person and the whole situation and what the needs are. Because what one person needs in 1005 is going to be totally different from a person with a similar diagnosis next door. And only the personal touch of a nurse, one who cares and one who's knowledgeable, can deliver that. I think that's where primary care is trying to get to on the floors. But it's just not there because the staffing is still not able to handle that. I think to do primary care, you can't have more than one or two patients and do it right, not in a facility like mine where the acuity is so high.

What are the biggest changes in critical care that you've seen since your first experience?

Oh, gosh, the technology, the acuity of the patients. We do so much more as nurses now. We do as much or more now as a nurse than the physicians did twenty years ago. I was around when the first Swan-Ganz catheters were introduced, and it was a really big deal. None of us knew what we were doing. The doctors had very specific parameters what we could do and what we couldn't, because we were not—we didn't have the medications, I don't think, at the time. We had Aramine and Levophed for blood pressure and that was about it. And those were life-or-death, dire situations when we used them. And the doctors would—you had to call them for every little thing, every little change. We would read Swan numbers but we didn't know what they meant. We just knew that if the wedge was above whatever we had to call somebody. But we didn't know what it meant. And, unfortunately, we didn't have the medications to treat things like we do now. So I think that's some of the biggest changes. I think the autonomy of nurses and the broadening scope of nursing has been a big change for the better. You don't see, when a doctor walks in the room if a nurse is doing something at the desk, she doesn't jump to her feet and offer her seat. She might say now, "Don't leave before I see you because I have some things that you need to do."

That's different.

It's totally different.

So how has nursing responded to all those changes?

I think more education. There are constant in-services.

In terms with what nurses do with patients?

Oh, what nurses do with patients. We're more involved in terms of teaching. At one time, this was early in my nursing career and until probably ten years ago, there was very little teaching that went on between the nurse and the patient. And up until ten to twelve, I can't even remember how many years ago, when the doctors wrote a prescription for a patient, the pharmacist didn't even put what that drug was, what the name of the drug was on the bottle. It was just, "Take this twice a day for cough or take this," or whatever. All of that patient education change has come into play, and patients are more knowledgeable. Nurses are far more knowledgeable. And instead of just responding to a doctor's order, we take those orders, interpret them, and do what needs to be done, not that we aren't following orders, but we have to know what's appropriate for that patient and what's not and know that doctors are human and can screw up too. And we can't—nurses are not blind followers anymore. We're leaders in a lot of ways, and I think on a much more collegial basis with the physician, especially some of the newer ones that are coming out of school now. I had a doctor, just recently we were putting in a line and he had disposed of all his sharps, had this nice neat tray, and was disassembling everything, had left everything neatly. I thanked him for it. I said, "This is great. You must be married to a nurse." He said, "No, I was raised by one." So I think we've come a long way in the eyes of the physicians. I think our status has improved. Is that a roundabout answer?

No, that helps. Do you see nurses leaving nursing?

I do, but not the extent that I used to. When I was 23, 24 years old, everybody I knew—every nurse I knew was my age. But we're all getting older now and we're all still doing it. Twenty years ago I never saw a nurse over 35 or

40 unless it was somebody who maybe had raised her kids and was gone and came back to it. You just didn't see older nurses. Everybody's goal was to get married, go home, and never come back. It wasn't a career, it was a job. It was a short-term situation until something better came along. That's why—when I went into it, I thought, well, I do this for a few years until something better comes along. It never has. I'm still waiting. But I think that that's been one of the biggest changes I've seen in the nurses, themselves, are they're much older, they're more educated, more assertive, and more willing to risk offending someone, offending the physician to get done what needs to get done. And I don't think that by and large we're intimidated like we used to be. And maybe that's age or orneriness. But education too. If you know what needs to be done and you know the best means to an end, why not do it? Why go around the world or pussyfoot around it if you can just get to it. And I think the nurse is in a better position to see what needs to be done.

Get back to George and Alice again. What was difficult for the nurses that did get close to him and were involved in his care? You talked about the hope and the expectation that he would get a heart and would get better. It was hard when he didn't. Was there some point that you should have maintained some objectivity?

I remember a quote. I think it was beautiful. It was talking about the difference in hope and wishes. And it said that wishes were something that you really don't expect to happen but you're glad when it does, but hope was something that you really had to be involved in, that you really had to put all your heart and soul into and that you had to risk a lot to hope. When you were wishing, you didn't risk anything, because the stakes were such that, if it happened it happened, but you really hadn't risked anything. But in hope, there's a lot of risk there, and you have to involve yourself, heart and soul, in that process. And I think with them, we hoped, it wasn't just a wish, we assumed that it would happen. Here was this guy who, he didn't smoke, he didn't drink, he was married to the same woman twenty years, he had a great family, he went to church, he had done all the right things, and it just wasn't meant for him to die, it shouldn't have happened. And it never occurred to me, it never occurred to me that he would die. It just never occurred to me until that last weekend when we put him on the balloon and he was so sick. It just never occurred to me that he would die. I thought that he would get better. Even until the last minute, even up until the hours before he died. Even though he had said he was never going to get a heart, we looked at that as, you know, like a kid, "It's never going to be my birthday," or, you know, "I'll never get that baseball bat that I want," kind of a negative because you can't see into the future. He never expected to get a heart. It was clear that he didn't. We thought that he would. And the only thing in retrospect that I think that we could have done differently is be more objective. But I don't know how you can do that.

Well, what would that have accomplished?

Yeah, exactly. It wouldn't have changed anything from a personal stand-point. Because if you detach yourself too much, you lose an awful lot of what nursing's all about. And I try to look at my patients, I try to treat them like I would want to be treated, and I want to treat them as whole people and not just the cardiomyopathy in room 1007. I want to be treated as a person with individual needs.

You don't get that involved with everybody?

No, because some—a lot of our patients are short-term, you've got them—and I work weekends; so you're there for a weekend, and then you're gone, and they're gone, and they've either gone to the floor, or home, or died, or whatever. But the—some people you just mesh with, you just hit it off with. And there have been a couple of patients over the past five years that I've really felt close to. And I found out this weekend that one of them had died. And I told the girl, I said, "Well, I can just quit nursing now. All my favorite patients are dead. There's nothing left for me." But I know there will be more, and I hope to make as much of an impact on their lives as they did mine, without being mushy. I've known nurses who just would fall all over somebody, but it's not real. And I think just being real people and being a friend first, and an advocate a close second, and a nurse maybe third. He would not have done well if we had gone in, "Hi, there. I'm your nurse. You will do things this way. You will eat when I tell you to. You will bathe when I tell you to." It wouldn't have worked with him. It didn't work with most people I've found. All of us want to have our own independence to the degree we can.

Do you think that kind of involved approach with patients protects you to some extent from burnout or does it make it harder? I look sometimes at the oncology doctors, I wonder how they do it. I mean, I don't know how you deal with people who die all the time.

I don't know either. You have to know your limitations and when you can dive in and when you can't.

But does it make it difficult to deal with inefficiency in the hospital setting and the lack of staffing?

It's real frustrating and I don't know whether it makes you better or more prone to burnout or less. Right. And I think you have to do things with all your heart and soul or they're not worth doing. And in terms of burnout, I think sometimes when I'm—when I am the most frustrated with nursing, then somebody like George comes along that restores your faith in the process, and even though he died, we made a difference, we made a big difference, and we were able to make the last four months of his life as normal and as productive as they could have been. We didn't treat him like an invalid. We didn't make him an invalid. He was able to maintain friendships and a family life of sorts.

A nurse told me one time that what nursing does is let patients set short-term goals and work with them to do it, like a pain-free afternoon is a reasonable goal.

Right. You don't have to get through it until Christmas or get all better, but a pain-free afternoon is something that a nurse can work toward and be happy with. Like that Kris Kristofferson song, "help me make it through the night"; sometimes that's the best you can hope for, is just get through one day at a time. But with the Donners, I just assumed they'd be there until he got the heart and we'd get the heart any minute. And that was kind of an exciting part of working weekends, because that's when I assumed the heart would come in. It just never came and I don't know why, still don't think it's fair. I need to talk to God about it when I get a chance.

Think about transplants. Do you think it's worth it, I mean, the hope? Is it a realistic hope? Do you think most people are pretty clear about what the reality on the other side could be?

No, I don't think most people have any idea what the other side's going to be. The other side of it is some people do well and some don't and some reject and get really sick and that kind of existence in the hospital is not a pretty sight, but by the time they get to us and they're on drips, it's a last-ditch effort, they're committed. And whether or not they want—whether or not they know what it's really like on the other side is irrelevant at that point.

It's either death or that.

Right. So, considering the options, you go for the best shot you got. And attitude is so important in survival too. Whether or not you—I'm a firm believer, I mean, if you expect good things, you're more likely to get them, you don't always. I think you've got a better shot at it than if you expect bad things, because you're likely to get what you expect there too. We had a guy with us a couple of months ago who was—it was just for the short term. He'd come in for a tune-up and he was a young man and went home, doing relatively well medically managed and got his call—we were leaving one Sunday night and he was coming through the ER, he was on a stretcher, and he was high as a kite, he was waving to everybody, he was going to get a heart, he was really happy. Well, he had a horrible post-op course. He was on the balloon, he was in and out of the unit, just a horrible time. He was having rejection problems, couldn't get him off the ventilator for weeks and weeks and weeks. Well, he's home now and doing fine, but it was a really rocky course, and he was only thirty-something, a young guy, didn't smoke, you know, had relatively low risk factors. But he sent some handmade goodies to the unit yesterday and he's doing fine. So now you can say it was worth it. But when he was going through it, we were thinking, oh, it's such a shame, he's such a nice guy and he was home, he was doing well on medical management, to come in and go through that living hell, not to mention the expense. But he's doing fine now. You don't know, it's a toss-up. The ones that you really think would be a great candidate, like the Donners. He had some antibodies from a blood transfusion from years before and he was—I think he was A negative. Plus, he was a big guy and he needed a bigger heart. They had even talked about piggyback. But because of his AICD and the problems he had with his arrhythmias, they didn't want to consider that. So he had a couple of strikes against him. But we just sort of poo-pooed those, "Na, he'll be all right." He seemed too nice a guy to die.

Well, what do you do to help?
You're committed, you're in for the duration.
How do nurses intervene in those kinds of situations?
I think, there again, advocates. They know what the patients are thinking more than a physician does. They've got the interaction with the family and the patient. I think life is sacred. I'm pro-life in terms of the abortion issue. But on the flip side, when you've got somebody that's terminal, I don't have a problem with allowing them to die with dignity either, not necessarily euthanasia, but allowing some withdrawal treatment for humanitarian reasons. I have a patient I took care of just last night who was dying. The family had a conditional code. They said we could not do compressions and we couldn't intubate, but we could give drugs and we could shock. I don't think families are necessarily in a position alone to make those decisions without some support and some information. The families will say, "I want everything done." But they don't know what everything is. Everything is horrible. And to let them kind of know what "everything" means and how long we can prolong this. Well, this lady last night, who probably has died by now, we could have done lots of things to intervene, but her underlying problem was she was 70 years old and had leukemia, and she's been sick since January and has not responded at all, and she's just gone downhill. But we could have—she had a good strong heart. We

could have intervened and intubated, put her on Levophed, done all sorts of things and kept her alive for weeks to come. But she's unconscious now; so what have we accomplished there. There's some tough decisions to make. And I think the nurses are in a better position to talk to the families, educate the families, and help them make the right decision or a decision they can live with. Because the doctors kind of flash in and out and they don't have the rapport that we have with them. And one of my pat answers, I guess, to patients' families, when the end is in sight and they start this, "Oh, well, I should of done this or I should have done that," or "Why didn't I take Mamma earlier or whatever," and I just tell them that, "You made the best decision with the information you had at the time and you can't feel guilty about it. You've done the best you can and you can't look back." And then you've seen deaths that were so good, people who made their decisions and were allowed to slip into a coma or whatever with the family around.

Nursing is pretty complex.

Yes, I think too, with the Donners, they were comfortable with their own mortality and immortality, they felt comfortable with their salvation and felt that he would just be going home. So, that—the death part wasn't as big an issue in terms of a fear as just not wanting to give up what you have here on earth. And I just think we all go through that.

I appreciate your talking to me about the Donners.

There is so much more emotion involved than I can conjure up, I guess, right now. There was so much that went on, just—it was losing a friend as well as a patient. And I felt kind of mixed feelings that I was so close to him. And the day that he needed the balloon pump, I was there—I was taking care of him. And I was involved in putting the balloon pump in on that Saturday. And then the following Saturday he died, the same thing, on my shift. And his wife said—this is really—it really touched me, she said, "He was waiting for you to come back so he could die, and he wanted to be with someone he could be comfortable with. He didn't want to die with strangers."

Was he alert up until the end?

We had sedated him the last few days of the week; so, by the time he actually died, no, he wasn't. He was on a Fentanyl drip, I think. But he wasn't unconscious, I guess. I mean, his wife would talk to him and hold his hand and she'd get a squeeze every now and then. He was pretty deep purposely. It was clear there was nothing left to do. He'd gotten septic by then and he was on maximum support, drips, balloon, ventilator. What could you do?

He was totally life support?

Yeah. But he just—he was a "no code" by then. But it went so fast. It just went so fast. I mean, you don't usually see somebody up walking down the halls one day and then a week later—

Is there any way to help people be prepared that they might not get a heart? Is there any way or is there any usefulness to that?

Yeah. We've had several patients who came in and obviously, in the beginning, had very unrealistic expectations. One man said—he came in and said, "Well, I'm here to get a heart. You think they've got one in my size?" I guess he thought that we just went to the utility room and pulled one off the shelf. These folks have had no education about it. And it seems like they're the ones that get their hearts in two days. And then you've got the folks that come in that are well prepared and educated and understand what they're in for, like the Donners. They had researched everything. He had recurring bouts of CHF [congestive heart failure] for a year and would come in for a couple of days and go home. So they knew what they were in for. They knew that this was it for the long haul. But you've got a lot of folks that don't. And I wonder what sort of information these guys are getting in their doctor's office, especially ones that come from another hospital. Now, I think the ones that come through this system have a pretty good idea, they must have some pretty good nurses. I give it to the nurses, not the physicians. But you get these folks that come in from outlying hospitals that are transferred to us for a work-up and they're the ones with the most unrealistic expectations. They expect to come in, get their heart, you know, "here one day, heart the next, and home the next week." And I don't think they're prepared for the wait and for the inevitability that, you know, it may never come, they may never get a heart. And then, you talk to people whose family members are waiting for transplants, and I've asked them, "Are you an organ donor, would you donate your organs?" And they say, "No." Just blows me away that they're there waiting for their loved one to get a heart, or a kidney, or whatever, but they themselves would never donate. But Mrs. Donner wore her little button about, "Don't take your organs with you to heaven." She was a big advocate and she went to all the support meetings. They did all the right things; so it shouldn't have happened that he died. I think that too is part of our bias, cultural bias or whatever. The people that do the right things, and if they're nice-looking and they're good people, then all should go well. But if you get—you know, you get somebody who's off the street, who's dabbled in drugs or whatever, no support systems, and then suddenly everything works out fine for them. I guess it's like the—you know, why good things happen to bad people. I read that book. I gave it to Mrs. Donner after he died. She's a great lady and she's doing fine.

I'm glad. That's interesting you've kept in touch with her.

Yeah, we've talked several times. She's a good lady. And she said that she would probably get married again but George would always be first. They had been married—they had been high school sweethearts and got married when she was—I think she was 18, he was 19, and had been married 20 years. They just had the twentieth-year, or were about to have a twentieth-year anniversary. That's a long time to be with one person. I didn't make it that long, and if I'm ever going to I better get started soon.

This view of the experiences of the practicing critical care nurse documented the personal characteristics and commitments of nurses to patients and nursing, the progression of a largely female occupational group, and the values of the larger society as health care has become complex, highly technical, and invasive. The values experienced in this study represent those of committed, motivated nurses who are still in practice settings. The realities of mediocrity, indifference, and burnout in nurses and physicians in critical care deserve the attention of scholars. This study portrays some of the diverse characteristics of critical care settings.

Nurses were the persistent human factor in the critical care settings described. They consistently expressed a commitment to patients and demonstrated the ability to assume highly complex and sophisticated patient care skills. The settings where critical care is practiced and the nature of patient care itself are stressful. These stresses and existing conflicts between the professional goals of nursing and the economic realities of the hospital as employer may further increase a serious shortage of nurses in the United States and internationally. While care has become increasingly complex, hospitals are "downsizing" and cutting nursing positions, both at the bedside and in support roles. Many nurses are reflecting on the personal costs of providing that care with fewer nurses in settings that are increasingly ambivalent to some of the aims of nursing.

Further, caring has been a traditionally feminine attribute. The ways in which nurses and nursing, hospitals, and the larger society value and define that caring may determine the existence or demise of nursing in the future. Patients in contemporary critical care settings are vulnerable and require nursing care. These settings will become even more complex. Nursing has not sufficiently defined and protected its scope of practice so that the critical elements of nursing care are assured. This leaves nursing and patients vulnerable to the economic priorities of for-profit groups.

The nurses interviewed expressed a high degree of commitment to patient care and a willingness to combine that with performance of expert skills. The goals of nursing seem congruent with the trends in health care that reflect consumer participation, prevention, health promotion, and a demand for institutional accountability. Nurses expressed commitment to such goals. The interpersonal contract between nurse and patient would seem the likely model for professional practice expressed by the nurses interviewed. Critical care nursing represents a model of professional and institutional practice that is unique at the present time. Critical care nursing may be able to translate that particular combination of competence and caring into formal power in the hospital setting for the good of nursing and for the humane and ethical care of patients.

Appendix

The purpose of this research was to acquire and interpret, through the techniques and methods of oral history, information from interviews with critical care nurses. Traditional histories of nursing cited chronology relative to major world events, and two biases were persistent. First, nursing was viewed in the shadow of the history of medicine and the uniqueness of nursing was absent in the telling of the story. Two examples illustrate this bias. Mark Hilberman, a physician, managed to describe the evolution of the intensive care unit with only incidental mention of nurses (1975). This is notable since the primary characteristic of any intensive care unit is the twenty-four-hour surveillance of patients by nurses. Paul Starr, a sociologist, scarcely mentioned nurses in his Pulitzer Prize-winning study of the rise of medicine and the health industry in the United States (1982). Yet nurses represent the largest group of health care workers in the United States.

Nurses as women generated the second bias in traditional histories. Nurses as individuals were as invisible as nursing has been as a discipline. Developments in social history over the past two decades, particularly those concerned with the experiences of women, racial and ethnic minorities, and workers have generated interest in the nurse's past, present, and future roles in health care. Interest in the study of nursing was generated from recognition of the nurse as "worker," as participant in a problematic hospital bureaucracy, as "female," and as part of the "history from below," or history of ordinary females, their ailments and treatments (Rosenberg, 1987: 67–68). Even when the stories of women and nurses have been addressed, the impact of specialization and regional influences may be absent. Further, while the details of nursing education and professional organization were well documented, the story of the development of actual clinical practice was almost non-existent. As a result, the elite leadership was documented while the hands-on practicing nurse was anonymous.

Finding primary source materials for recreating the experience of the practicing nurse may be problematic. First, practicing nurses are unlikely to have left formal papers to be preserved in archives. Second, the few written records that may exist are not likely to address the heart of the nurse's human interactions with birth, death, illness, and critical life events, although selected autobiographies of nurses do exist and reflect this quality of human experience in certain circumstances. Third, technological developments in communication like the telephone and the computer have replaced the traditional source materials of personal letters and diaries. Finally, much of the research about nursing behaviors has been quantitative in methodology and may not reflect the subtleties and complexities of human interaction, and the image of nursing practice is incomplete. "The quality of historical scholarship rests on its ability to assemble the best facts and generate the most cogent explanation of a given situation or period" (Lynaugh and Reverby, 1987: 4). The personal story of the practicing nurse represents an integral part of the history of the profession.

David Dunaway and Willa Baum (1984: xiii–xvii) have described three phases of oral history in the United States. The pioneering works of Allan Nevins and Louis Starr at Columbia University during the 1940s defined the first phase, which viewed oral methods as significant tools for biography and autobiography and as source materials for generations of future historians. The second phase reflected the social activism of the 1960s. Oral history came to be viewed as more than a collection of non-traditional sources. The techniques were used to empower non-literate, ethnically diverse, and underrepresented groups. Oral history collections grew during this period, and the Oral History Association was formalized (*Oral History: Evaluation Guidelines,* 1980). The third phase reflected a more mature discipline, concerned with interviews as history and with issues of technology, public use of oral methods, archival collections, and interdisciplinary approaches to popular history, culture, and language. Oral history methods also became more visible to the public as a result of project sponsorship by the Public Broadcasting Association, the National Endowment for the Humanities, and other policy-making and funding groups.

Oral methods have been used by many disciplines, including history, sociology, political science, cultural anthropology, and psychology (Abzug, 1985; Bellah et al., 1985; Hall, Korstad, and Leloudis, 1986). Oral tradition has been viewed as an acceptable substitute for the written record, as an art form representing particular culture and time, and as a unique expression of human dimensions not readily found in written records. Robert Abzug used oral interviews with concentration camp liberators to tell the American military experience of liberation. He described their import: "They afford us a window on the way men and women act and think when faced with the unimaginable suffering of others. The deep compassion and sometimes the limits of vision displayed . . . pointed to important ambivalences about facing the Holocaust and its victims . . . and the immediate and long-range impact of their discoveries on the public mind" (Abzug, 1985: xi).

It is this last characteristic that made oral interviews with critical care nurses an appropriate method for the present study. Written records, even if they existed, were an inappropriate source to reflect the heart of the nurses' experience with human suffering. The strengths and limitations of self-reporting as valid source material for scholarly writing have been identified. T. Lummis identifies two criteria for validity of oral evidence: first, the degree to which any individual interview yields accurate information, and, second, the degree to which the individual interview is representative of its time and place (Lummis, 1981: 109; Mitchell, 1983: 285; Polit and Hungler, 1991: 277–300).

In 1980 the Oral History Association proposed project evaluation guidelines for the production and use of oral history, "especially the principles, rights and obligation for the creation of source material that is authentic, useful and reliable" (*Oral History: Evaluation Guidelines,* 1980: 3). These guidelines have been used in designing this study to ensure project integrity and protection of human rights.

Methodology

Three forms were developed for conducting the study. The Informed Consent and Release Agreement, designed to conform to the Oral History Association Guidelines, explained the purpose of the research project, the conditions of the exchange, and the uses to be made of the taped interview material. Care was taken to make sure each interviewee fully understood the agreement before participating. To maintain anonymity, pseudonyms were randomly selected from the Atlanta telephone directory.

The Personal Data Form, covering personal and professional background data, was completed before the interview was conducted. The information gathered was used (1) to cue the interview itself about particular background issues relevant to the interview questions; and (2) to compile the general description of the characteristics of the group. A summary of this information is included below.

The Interview Schedule followed during the interviews themselves was developed around five major headings reflecting the purposes of the study and the information obtained from the literature about critical care nursing. First, I asked for an overall sketch of the nurse's life. This provided an opportunity for me to establish priorities and focus. It also provided information about the motivation for the meaning of nursing as an occupation. This less structured interchange allowed for a degree of interpersonal comfort, trust, and intimacy to develop prior to the goal-directed questions. The interview began with an introduction to the attitudes and values of the nurse interviewee. The remaining section contained open-ended questions about nursing education, nursing practice, technology, and ethical dimensions of practice. I asked for specific clinical examples and personal experiences as a part of the interview process. The structured interview was piloted in two interviews and revised. Forms developed for the study were presented in the original dissertation or may be obtained from the author.

Twenty-five interviews were conducted. The interviews were taped, using broadcast quality audiocassette tape and recording equipment, and transcribed. The transcripts were reviewed for content analysis, and selected portions were included in the body of the written work. Editing consisted of removing extraneous words ("ah," "um," and the like) and telephone interruptions, using pseudonyms for real patients, and removing references to specific places; no attempt was made to correct grammar, delete expletives, or paraphrase. The uniqueness of each nurse's story and style reflected as much about the person and the nurse as the words that were spoken.

The tapes were compared to the transcripts to assure accuracy. Since these are not to be a permanent collection, the interviewees did not review the transcripts for accuracy.

The primary criterion for selection of a sample population is representativeness (Polit and Hungler, 1991: 253–273). I selected the nurse participants from the critical care nurse population in Atlanta. This sample is considered unbiased and representative of the larger population of critical care nurses because of several factors. First, the national standards of critical care practice and education described in Chapter 1 are promoted by the American Association of Critical Care Nursing, the Joint Commission on Accreditation of Healthcare Organizations, and the Georgia State Board of Nursing. Second, all participants are registered nurses (RNs) with critical care experience. Third, further measures were taken to reduce sample bias, including selection of twenty-five participants who represented a range of critical care experiences. Participants were selected to represent experience in critical care settings over time from the 1950s until the present; work in rural and urban areas, in teaching and private hospitals, and in military and VA and non-military hospitals; and diversity in age, race, educational background, and range of staff management and clinical experiences in hospitals. An effort was made to include participants not known personally to me to reduce biases of preconceptions. The structured interview guide further limited this bias. Table 2 presents the results of the sample in a manner that will protect the privacy of the participants.

Finally, I am a nurse, with twenty years of experience in nursing education and practice, including critical care nursing. My life experience parallels many of the developments in critical care discussed in this book. This fact might be considered an enhancement as well as a bias. The efforts to insure objectivity described above may well limit potential bias. Many of the interviews were quite powerful and intimate and almost cathartic. My impression that for many of the nurses this was the first opportunity to express so much about themselves and nursing in such a personal way was borne out by the concurrence of several nurses. I repeatedly experienced this sense of intimacy and power as the twenty-five interviews were conducted. Several explanations are plausible. Perhaps this response represents a characteristic of oral history methods, especially in interviews dealing with issues of life experience, commitment, and compassion. Susan Reverby, a non-nurse historian of women's issues and nursing, has noted that she is inevitably asked whether she, her parents, or her husband are nurses or in medicine. She attributes this question to nursing's supposed unimportance except to those in the field and to a pervasive sexism (1987: xi). The characteristics of individuals, primarily women, who have traditionally become nurses, and the complex interplay of the art and science and work of nursing, may also explain this phenomenon.

The colloquial nature of the interpersonal exchange in the interviews sometimes uses almost poetic descriptions of meaningful human intimacies. It also reflects the argot of an occupational group. In particular, the nurses consistently used the pronoun "she" for nurses and "he" for both physicians and patients. As noted earlier, the interviews are included essentially verbatim in the text. An effort has been made to preserve the conversational tenor of the interviews, as well as the individuality and character of each nurse, by retaining the actual words of the speakers, with no effort to "rewrite" or "correct" them. Questions by the interviewer are set in darker type. Explanations of technical language and occupational argot have been bracketed for the non-nurse reader.

TABLE 2   Characteristics of the Sample of Twenty-Five Critical Care Nurses

Personal

Age (27–61)		*Sex*		*Religion*	
27–29	1	Female	24	Protestant	18
30–34	8	Male	1	Catholic	5
35–39	6			Pentecostal	1
40–44	5	*Race*			
45–49	0	Caucasian	21		
50–54	1	Black	4		
55–59	2				
60–64	2				

Marital status (number of children)

Single	11	(one has 1 child)
Married	5	(one has 2 children)
Divorced	8	(one with 3 children, one with 2, three with 1)
Widowed	1	(no children)

Professional

First degree (highest degree)

Diploma in nursing	11	(dip, 1; BS, 1; BA, 1; BSN, 1; MN, 6; PhD, 1)
Associate degree	2	(AD, 1; MN, 1)
BSN	12	(BSN, 2; MN, 9; PhD, 1)

Year of graduation (years in nursing)

1947–60	5	(27–40)
1965–72	7	(15–22)
1973–76	6	(11–14)
1977–87	7	(7–10)

States of practice or education: Alabama, Delaware, District of Columbia, Florida, Georgia, Illinois, Indiana, Louisiana, Maryland, Michigan, Mississippi, New Jersey, New York, North Carolina, Ohio, Oklahoma, Pennsylvania, South Carolina, Virginia, Washington

Professional certification

CCRN (critical care)	11
CNOR (operating room)	1
ACLS (advanced cardiac life support, AHA)	3

TABLE 2   (*Continued*)

Professional memberships

American Association of Critical Care Nursing	15
American Nurses' Association (Georgia Nurses' Association)	12
National League for Nursing	2
Sigma Theta Tau (National Honor Society for Nursing)	6
Other associations (operating room, rehabilitation, business, gerontology, surgery)	7

*Range of experience**

Clinical (non-critical care): cardiology, clinical instruction, diabetes treatment, medical-surgical, oncology, psychiatry, rehabilitation

Clinical (critical care): cardiovascular ICU, coronary care unit, ICU, ICU float pool, operating room, orthopedics/neuro ICU, pediatric open heart ICU, recovery room, renal/burn ICU, trauma ICU

Administrative (hospital): head nurse; nursing administration

Education: university faculty

Current position: staff nurse (CCU, ICU, surgical ICU, open-heart ICU); clinical specialist (cardiology, surgery); head nurse; assistant director of nursing; clinical coordinator; graduate nursing student

*No attempt is made to present a quantitative range. The purpose of these categories is to portray the range of experiences that characterize the sample population.

Clearly, one sample bias is persistent. This sample represented the nurses still employed in nursing in critical care settings. These participants were willing to be interviewed and motivated to talk about their experiences in critical care. Since graduation, they have all been continuously employed in nursing or pursuing nursing education. The results of this study will, therefore, more likely represent the committed, motivated nurse, and the critical care nurse able to cope with the complexities of the setting, than the total population of critical care nurses through the evolution of critical care. The sample omits those nurses who have left nursing or critical care settings and those unwilling to be interviewed. Increasing complexities in critical care nursing and the impact of the nursing shortage and efforts to relieve it will also require further study.

The strength of the sample population is its representativeness. The twenty-five nurses had a wide range of experience and education in many areas of the United States. The collective impressions reveal much about the commonalities of their experience in critical care settings. The current experiences of the nurses interviewed are in the South, so particular regional characteristics and contrasts may be possible.

The limitations of the sample relate to the size of the sample and the limited representation from particular groups (males, Hispanics, Asians, and other minorities). Further research should utilize this pilot study as a data base and focus attention on specific groups and characteristics, possibly including males, Blacks, and other minorities, regional groups, and particular types of units, hospitals, or experiences during war, crisis, hostage taking, disasters, and the like.

References

Abramson, Norman S. et al. (1980). "Adverse Occurrences in Intensive Care Units." *Journal of the American Medical Association* 244(14): 1582–1584.

Abzug, Robert H. (1985). *Inside the Vicious Heart: Americans and the Liberation of the Nazi Concentration Camps*. New York: Oxford University Press.

Ad Hoc Committee of the Harvard Medical School (1968). "A Definition of Irreversible Coma." *Journal of the American Medical Association* 205(6): 337–340.

Aiken, Linda H. (1990). "Charting the Future of Hospital Nursing." *Image* 22(2): 72–78.

Alspach, JoAnn Grif and Susan M. Williams (1991). *Core Curriculum for Critical Care Nursing*. 4th ed. Philadelphia: W. B. Saunders.

American Association of Critical Care Nurses (1984). *Definition of Critical Care Nursing*. Newport Beach, Calif.: AACN.

—— Position Statement (1987). *The Critical Care Clinical Nurse Specialist: Role Definition*. Newport Beach, Calif.: AACN.

—— (1990). *AACN Position Statement on Withholding and/or Withdrawal of Life-Sustaining Treatment*. Newport Beach, Calif.: AACN.

American Nurses' Association (1973). *Standards of Clinical Nursing Practice*. Kansas City, Mo.: AMA.

—— (1980). *Nursing, a Social Policy Statement*. Kansas City, Mo.: ANA.

—— (1985). *ANA Code for Nurses*. Kansas City, Mo.: ANA.

——, Committee on Ethics (1988). "Withdrawing or Withholding Food and Fluid." *American Journal of Nursing* 88(6): 797–801.

AMH 79: Accreditation Manual for Hospitals (1979). Chicago: Joint Commission on Accreditation of Hospitals.

AMH 87: Accreditation Manual for Hospitals (1987). Chicago: Joint Commission on Accreditation of Hospitals.

AMH: Accreditation Manual for Hospitals (1992). Oakbrook Terrace, Ill.: Joint Commission on Accreditation of Healthcare Organizations.

"An Appraisal of the Criteria of Cerebral Death" (1977). *Journal of the American Medical Association* 237 (10): 982–986.

Ayres, Stephen M. (1984). "Introduction: Critical Care Medicine." In Joseph E. Parillo and Stephen M. Ayres, eds., *Major Issues in Critical Care Medicine*. Baltimore: Williams and Wilkins.

Bailey, John T., Duane Walker, and Nancy Madsen (1980). "The Design of Stress Management Program for Stanford Intensive Care Nurses." *Journal of Nursing Education* 19(6): 26–24.

Bandman, Elsie L. and Bertram Bandman (1990). *Nursing Ethics Through the Life Span*. 2nd ed. Norwalk, Conn.: Appleton and Lange.

Beardsley, J. Murray, J. Robert Bowen, and Carmine J. Capalbo (1956). "Centralized Treatment for Seriously Ill Surgical Patients." *Journal of the American Medical Association* 162(6): 544–547.

Beauchamp, Tom C. and Leroy Walter, eds. (1989). *Contemporary Issues in Bioethics.* 3rd ed. Belmont, Calif.: Wadsworth Publishing.

Bellah, Robert N., Richard Madsen, William M. Sullivan, Ann Swidler, and Stephen Tipton (1985). *Habits of the Heart: Individualism and Commitment in American Life.* Berkeley and Los Angeles: University of California Press.

Benjamin, Martin and Joy Curtis (1992). *Ethics in Nursing.* 3rd ed. New York: Oxford University Press.

Benner, Patricia E. (1984). *From Novice to Expert: Excellence and Power in Clinical Nursing Practice.* Menlo Park, Calif.: Addison-Wesley.

Benner, Patricia E. and Judith Wrubel (1989). *The Primacy of Caring: Stress and Coping in Health and Illness.* Menlo Park, Calif.: Addison-Wesley.

Bennett, Ivan L., Jr. (1977). "Technology as a Shaping Force." *Daedalus* 106(1): 125–133.

Bilodeau, Carolyn Basio (1973). "The Nurse and Her Reactions to Critical Care Nursing." *Heart and Lung* 2(3): 358–362.

Birckhead, Loretta M. (1978). "Nursing and the Technetronic Age." *Journal of Nursing Administration* 8(2): 16–19.

Black, Henry Campbell (1968). *Black's Law Dictionary.* 4th ed. St. Paul, Minn.: West Publishing Company.

—— (1979). *Black's Law Dictionary.* 5th ed. St. Paul, Minn.: West Publishing Company.

—— (1990). *Black's Law Dictionary.* 6th ed. St. Paul, Minn.: West Publishing Company.

Blackburn, Susan (1982). "The Neonatal ICU: A High-Risk Environment." *American Journal of Nursing* 82(11): 1708–1712.

Bloom, Allan (1987). *The Closing of the American Mind.* New York: Simon and Schuster.

Bolter, J. David (1984). *Turing's Man: Western Culture in the Computer Age.* Chapel Hill: University of North Carolina Press.

Bresnahan, James F. (1987). "Suffering and Dying Under Intensive Care: Ethical Disputes Before the Courts." *Critical Care Nursing Quarterly* 10(2): 11–16.

Brown, Esther Lucille (1948). *Nursing for the Future.* New York: Russell Sage Foundation.

—— (1970). *Nursing Reconsidered: A Study of Change. Part I: The Professional Role in Institutional Nursing.* Philadelphia: J. B. Lippincott.

Bruhn, John G. (1978). "The Doctor's Touch: Tactile Communication in the Doctor-Patient Relationship." *Southern Medical Journal* 71(12): 1469–1473.

Brunt, J. Howard (1985). "An Exploration of the Relationship Between Nurses' Empathy and Technology. *Nursing Administration Quarterly* 9(4): 69–78.

Cahill, Sharon B. and Marytherese Balskus, eds. (1986). *Intervention in Emergency Nursing: The First 60 Minutes.* Rockville, Md.: Aspen Systems.

Callahan, Daniel (1977). "Health and Society: Some Ethical Imperatives." *Daedalus* 106(1): 23–34.

Campbell, Margaret L. and Richard W. Carlson (1992). "Terminal Weaning From Mechanical Ventilation: Ethical and Practical Considerations For Patient Management." *American Journal of Critical Care* 1(3): 52–56.

Caplin, Marcy S. and Dorothy L. Sexton (1988). "Stresses Experienced by Spouses of Patients in a Coronary Care Unit with Myocardial Infarction." *Focus on Critical Care* 15(5): 31–40.

Capra, Fritzof (1982). *The Turning Point: Science, Society, and the Rising Culture.* New York: Simon and Schuster.

Carnevali, Doris L. (1985). "Nursing Perspectives in Health Care Technology." *Nursing Administration Quarterly* 9(4): 10–18.

Cauwels, Janice M. (1986). *The Body Shop: Bionic Revolutions in Medicine.* St. Louis: C. V. Mosby.

Chinn, Peggy L., ed. (1986). *Ethical Issues in Nursing.* Rockville, Md.: Aspen Systems.

Clark, E. Culpepper, Michael J. Hyde, and Eva M. McMahan (1980). "Communication in the Oral History Interview: Investigating Problems of Interpreting Oral Data." *International Journal of Oral History* 1(1): 28–40.

Cockshut, A. O. J. (1974). *Truth to Life: The Art of Biography in the Nineteenth Century.* New York: Harcourt Brace, Jovanovich.

Cohen, Frances, and Richard S. Lazarus (1983). "Coping and Adaptation in Health and Illness." In David Mechanic, ed., *Handbook on Health, Health Care, and the Health Professions.* New York: Free Press, 608–635.

Corwin, Ronald G. (1967). "The Professional Employee: A Study of Conflict in Nursing Roles." In Mark Abrahamson, ed., *The Professional in the Organization.* Chicago: Rand McNally, 93–102.

Cousins, Norman (1979). *Anatomy of an Illness as Perceived by the Patient: Reflections on Healing and Regeneration.* New York: W. W. Norton.

Cowart, Marie E., and Rodney F. Allen (1981). *Changing Conceptions of Health Care: Public Policy and Ethical Issues for Nurses.* Thorofare, N.J.: Charles B. Slack.

Cronin-Stubbs, Diane and Carol Ann Rooks (1985). "The Stress, Social Support, and Burnout of Critical Care Nurses: The Results of Research." *Heart and Lung* 14(1): 31–39.

Curtin, Leah and M. Josephine Flaherty (1982). *Nursing Ethics: Theories and Pragmatics.* Bowie, Md.: Robert J. Brady.

Daly, Barbara J., Barbara Newlon, Hugo D. Montenegro, and Terry Langdon (1993). "Withdrawal of Mechanical Ventilation: Ethical Principles and Guidelines for Terminal Weaning." *American Journal of Critical Care* 2(3): 217–223.

Davis, Anne J. and Mila J. Aroskar (1991). *Ethical Dilemmas and Nursing Practice.* 3rd ed. Norwalk, Conn.: Appleton and Lange.

Davison, Richard and Lisette Glusberg Davison (1987). "Medical Experimentation: Ethics in High Technology." *Critical Care Nursing Quarterly* 10(2): 29–36.

DeCrosta, Tony (1985). "MegaTrends in Nursing." *Nursing Life* 1: 17–21.

DeVisser, Pamela A. (1981). "The Effects of Technology on Critical Care Nursing Practice." *Focus on Critical Care* 7(4): 26–29.

Disch, Joanne (1981). "Survey of Critical Care Nursing Practice. Part I: Characteristics of Hospitals with Critical Care Units." *Heart and Lung* 10(6): 1047–1050.

Dixon, Elizabeth I. and James V. Mink, eds. (1967). *Oral History at Arrowhead: The Proceedings of the First National Colloquium on Oral History*. Los Angeles: Oral History Association.

"Doing Better and Feeling Worse: Health in the United States" (1977). *Daedalus* 106(1).

Douglass, Laura Mae and Ena Olivia Bevis (1983). *Nursing Management and Leadership in Action*. 4th ed. St. Louis: C. V. Mosby.

"The Dracula of Medical Technology" (1988). Editorial. *New York Times*. May 16, p. A16.

Dunaway, David K. and Willa K. Baum (1984). *Oral History: An Interdisciplinary Anthology*. Nashville, Tenn.: American Association for State and Local History/Oral History Association.

Elpern, Ellen H., Suzanne B. Yellen, and Laural A. Burton (1993). "A Preliminary Investigation of Opinions and Behaviors Regarding Advance Directives for Medical Care." *American Journal of Critical Care* 2(2): 161–167.

Fairman, Julie (1992). "Watchful Vigilance: Nursing Care, Technology, and the Development of Intensive Care Units." *Nursing Research* 41(1): 56–59.

Farrell, Barbara (1987). "AIDS Patients: Values in Conflict." *Critical Care Nursing Quarterly* 10(2): 74–85.

Fife, Betsy L. (1985). "A Model for Predicting the Adaptation of Families to Medical Crisis: An Analysis of Role Integration." *Image* 17(4): 108–112.

Flanagan, Lyndia, comp. (1976). *One Strong Voice: The Story of the American Nurses' Association*. Kansas City, Mo.: American Nurses' Association.

Freeman, Howard E., Robert J. Blendon, Linda H. Aiken, Seymour Sudman, Connie F. Mullinix, and Christopher R. Corey (1987). "Americans Report on Their Access to Health Care." *Health Affairs* 6(1): 6–18.

Friedman, Ernest H. (1972). "Stress and Intensive Care Nursing." *Heart and Lung* 1(6): 753–754.

—— (1982). "Stress and Intensive Care Nursing: A Ten Year Reappraisal." *Heart and Lung* 11(1): 26–28.

Gadow, Sally (1989). "Clinical Subjectivity: Advocacy with Silent Patients." *Nursing Clinics of North America* 24(2): 535–541.

Gardam, James E. D. (1969). "Nursing Stresses in the Intensive Care Unit." Letter. *Journal of the American Medical Association* 208(12): 2337–2338.

Garlo, Dolores M. (1984). "Critical Care Nurses: A Case for Legal Recognition of the Growing Responsibilities and Accountability in the Nursing Profession." *Journal of Contemporary Law* 11(1): 239–285.

Garraty, John A. (1957). *The Nature of Biography*. New York: Alfred A. Knopf.

Georgia Board of Nursing (1990). *Georgia Registered Professional Nurse Practice Act*. Atlanta: Georgia Department of State.

Georgia Nurses' Association, Nursing Shortage Task Force (1988). *An Historical Perspective of Federal Action Relative to Nursing*. Appendix B. Atlanta: GNA. (Courtesy of Emily Ellis).

Grady, Christine (1989). "Ethical Issues in Providing Nursing Care to Human

Immunodeficiency Virus-Infected Populations." *Nursing Clinics of North America* 24(2): 523–524.

Grele, Ronald J. (1975). "A Surmisable Variety: Interdisciplinarity and Oral Testimony. *American Quarterly* 27(3): 275–295.

—— (1985). *Envelopes of Sound: The Art of Oral History.* 2nd ed., rev. & enl. Chicago: Precedent Publishing.

Grob, Gerald (1977). "The Social History of Medicine and Disease in America: Problems and Possibilities." *Journal of Social History* 10(4): 391–409.

Hall, Jacquelyn David, Robert Korstad, and James Leloudis (1986). "Cotton Mill People: Work, Community, and Protest in the Textile South, 1880–1940." *American Historical Review* 91(2): 245–286.

Hall, Richard H. (1991). *Organizations: Structures, Process, and Outcomes.* 5th ed. Englewood Cliffs, N.J.: Prentice-Hall.

Halm, Margo A. and Michele A. Alpen (1993). "The Impact of Technology on Patients and Families." *Nursing Clinics of North America* 28(2): 443–457.

Harmer, Bertha and Virginia Henderson (1955). *Textbook of the Principles and Practice of Nursing.* 5th ed. New York: Macmillan.

Harris, Barbara J. (1978). *Beyond Her Sphere: Women and the Professions in American History.* Westport, Conn.: Greenwood Press.

Harrison, Margaret and Patricia H. Cotanch (1987). "Pain: Advances and Issues in Critical Care." *Nursing Clinics of North America* 22(3): 691–697.

Hay, Donald and Donald Oken (1972). "The Psychological Stresses of Intensive Care Nursing." *Psychosomatic Medicine* 34(2): 109–118.

Headlines Editor (1993). "A Law That Barred RNs from Giving Injections." *American Journal of Nursing* 93(3): 9.

Helton, Mary C., Susan H. Gordon, and Susan L. Nunnery (1980). "The Correlation Between Sleep Deprivation and the Intensive Care Unit Syndrome." *Heart and Lung* 9(3): 464–468.

Henderson, Deborah J. (1988). "HIV Infection: Risks to Health Care Workers and Infection Control." *Nursing Clinics of North America* 23(4): 767–777.

Henderson, Virginia (1961). *Basic Principles of Nursing Care.* London: International Council of Nurses.

—— (1985). "The Essence of Nursing in High Technology." *Nursing Administration Quarterly* 9(4): 1–9.

Henderson, Virginia and Gladys Nite (1978). *Principles and Practice of Nursing.* 6th ed. New York: Macmillan.

Hilberman, Mark (1975). "The Evolution of Intensive Care Units." *Critical Care Medicine* 3(4): 159–165.

Holloway, Nancy Meyer (1988). *Nursing the Critically Ill Adult.* 3rd ed. Menlo Park, Calif.: Addison-Wesley.

—— (1993). *Nursing the Critically Ill Adult.* 4th ed. Menlo Park, Calif.: Addison-Wesley.

Holsclaw, Pamela A. (1965). "Nursing in High Emotional Risk Areas." *Nursing Forum* 4(4): 36–45.

Hospital Survey Profile 1979 Edition (1979). Chicago: Joint Commission on Accreditation of Hospitals.

Hudak, Carolyn M., Thelma Lohr, and Barbara M. Gallo (1986). *Critical Care Nursing.* 3rd ed. Philadelphia: J. B. Lippincott.

Hudak, Carolyn M., Barbara M. Gallo, and Thelma Lohr (1990). *Critical Care Nursing: A Holistic Approach.* 5th ed. Philadelphia: J. B. Lippincott.

In re Quinlan (1975). 137, N.J. Sup. 227, 348 A.2d 801 (Ch. Div. 1975), *rev'd* 70 N.J. 10, 355 A.2d 647 (1976).

Jacobson, Sharol P. (1978). "Stressful Situations for Neonatal Intensive Care Nurses." *MCN: American Journal of Maternal Child Nursing* 3(3): 144–150.

Janis, Irving L. (1958). *Psychological Stress: Psychoanalytic and Behavioral Studies of Surgical Patients.* New York: John Wiley and Sons.

Jezewski, Mary Ann, Yvonne Sherer, Colleen Miller, and Ellen Battista (1993). "Consenting to DNR: Critical Care Nurses' Interactions with Patients and Family Members." *American Journal of Critical Care* 2(4): 302–309.

Kalisch, Philip Arthur and Beatrice J. Kalisch (1986). *The Advance of American Nursing.* 2nd ed. Boston: Little-Brown.

Kenner, Cornelia V., Cathie E. Guzzetti, and Barbara Montgomery Dossy (1985). *Critical Care Nursing: Body, Mind, Spirit.* 2nd ed. Boston: Little Brown.

Ketefian, Shake (1989). "Moral Reasoning and Ethical Practice in Nursing: Measurement Issues." *Nursing Clinics of North America* 24(2): 509–521.

Kieffer, George H. (1979). *Bioethics: A Textbook of Issues.* Reading, Mass.: Addison Wesley.

King, Shirley L. and Francis M. Gregor (1985). "Stress and Coping in Families of the Critically Ill." *Critical Care Nurse* 5(4): 48–51.

Kinney, Marguerite Rogers (1981). "Survey of Critical Care Nursing Practice. Part II: Unit Characteristics." *Heart and Lung* 10(6): 1051–1054.

Kinney, Marguerite Rogers, Donna R. Packa, and Sandra B. Dunbar (1993). *AACN's Clinical Reference for Critical Care Nursing.* 3rd ed. New York: McGraw-Hill.

Knox, Linda S. (1989). "Ethical Issues in Nutritional Support Nursing." *Nursing Clinics of North America* 24(2): 427–436.

Kornfield, Donald S., Teresita Maxwell, and Dawn Momrows (1968). "Psychological Hazards of the Intensive Care Unit." *Nursing Clinics of North America* 3(3): 41–51.

Koumans, Alfred J. R. (1965). "Psychiatric Consultation in an Intensive Care Unit." *Journal of the American Medical Association* 194(6): 133–137.

Kramer, Marlene (1974). *Reality Shock: Why Nurses Leave Nursing.* St. Louis: C. V. Mosby.

Krekeler, Kathleen (1987). "Critical Care Nursing and Moral Development." *Critical Care Nursing Quarterly* 10(2): 1–10.

Lewandowski, Wendy, Barbara Daly, Donna K. McClish, Barbara W. Juknialis, and Stuart J. Youngner (1985). "Treatment and Care of 'Do Not Resuscitate' Patients in a Medical Intensive Care Unit." *Heart and Lung* 14(2): 175–181.

Lisson, Edwin L. (1987). "Ethical Issues Related to Pain Control." *Nursing Clinics of North America* 22(3): 649–659.

Lummis, Trevor (1981). "Structure and Validity in Oral Evidence." *International Journal of Oral History* 2(2): 109–120.

Lumpp, Francesca (1979). "The Role of the Nurse in the Bioethical Decision-Making Process." *Nursing Clinics of North America* 14(1): 13–21.

Lynaugh, Joan E. and Julie Fairman (1992). "New Nurses, New Spaces: A Preview of the AACN History Study." *American Journal of Critical Care* 1(1): 19–24.

Lynaugh, Joan E. and Susan Reverby (1987). "Thoughts on the Nature of History." *Nursing Research* 36(1): 4, 69.

Lynn, Kenneth S., ed. (1965). *The Professions in America*. Boston: Houghton Mifflin.

Marlow, Dorothy R. (1977). *Textbook of Pediatric Nursing*. 5th ed. Philadelphia: W. B. Saunders.

Marlow, Dorothy R. and Barbara A. Redding (1988). *Textbook of Pediatric Nursing*. 6th ed. Philadelphia: W. B. Saunders.

Marriner, Ann, ed. (1979). *Current Perspectives in Nursing Management*. St. Louis: C. V. Mosley.

Martin, Darlene (1985). "Withholding Treatment from Severely Handicapped Newborns: Ethical-Legal Issues." *Nursing Administration Quarterly* 9(4): 47–56.

Martino, Joseph Paul (1993). *Technological Forecasting for Decision-Making*. 3rd ed. New York: McGraw-Hill.

Mathies, Allen W., Jr. (1978). "The Impact of New Life-Support Methodology on Medical Education and Practice." In Max Harry Weil and Robert S. Henning, eds., *Handbook of Critical Care Medicine*. Miami, Fla.: Symposium Specialists, 3–7.

May, William F. (1972). "The Sacral Power of Death in Contemporary Experience." *Social Research* 39(3): 463–488.

McCaman, Barbara and Harold L. Hirsh (1979). "Brain Death: Legal Issues." *Heart and Lung* 8(6): 1098–1102.

McDermott, Walsh (1977). "Evaluating the Physician and His Technology." *Daedalus* 106(1): 135–157.

Mead, Margaret (1956). "Nursing — Primitive and Civilized." *American Journal of Nursing* 56(8): 1001–1004.

Melosh, Barbara (1982). *The Physician's Hand: Work, Culture, and Conflict in American Nursing*. Philadelphia: Temple University Press.

Menard, Shirley W., ed. (1987). *The Clinical Nurse Specialist: Perspectives on Practice*. New York: John Wiley and Sons.

Menzies, Isabel E. P. (1960). "Nurses Under Stress." *International Nursing Review* 7(6): 9–16.

Miles, Steven H., Ronald Cranford, and Alvin L. Shultz (1982). "The Do-Not-Resuscitate Order in a Teaching Hospital." *Annals of Internal Medicine* 96(5): 660–663.

Mitchell, Pamela H., Litthe Habermann, Frankie Johnson, Deb Vanlwegren-Scott, and Donald Tyler (1985). "Critically Ill Children: The Importance of Touch in a High Technology Environment." *Nursing Administration Quarterly* 9(4): 38–46.

Moorhouse, Mary Frances, Alice C. Geissler, and Marilynn E. Doenges (1987). *Critical Care Plans: Guidelines for Patient Care*. Philadelphia: F. A. Davis.

Moos, Rudolf H. (1984). *Coping with Physical Illness*. New York: Plenum Medical Book Company.

Mumford, Lewis (1934). *Technics and Civilization*. New York: Harcourt Brace, Jovanovich.

Munch, Julia (1972). "Symposium on Units for Special Care: Foreword." *Nursing Clinics of North America* 7(2): 311–312.

Naisbitt, John (1982). *Megatrends: Ten New Directions Transforming Our Lives*. New York: Warner Books.

Neff, Walter Scott (1985). *Work and Human Behavior*. 3rd ed. Chicago: Aldine Publishers.

Neverschwander, John A. (1976). *Oral History as a Teaching Approach*. Washington, D.C.: National Education Association.

Nightingale, Florence (1859). *Notes on Nursing: What It Is and What It Is Not*. London: Harrison and Sons.

Noble, M. A., ed. (1982). *The ICU Environment: Directions for Nursing*. Reston, Va.: Reston Publishers.

Oberst, Marilyn T. (1986). "Nursing in the Year 2000: Setting the Agenda for Knowledge Generation and Utilization." In Gladys E. Sorensen, ed., *Setting the Agenda for the Year 2000: Knowledge Development in Nursing*. Kansas City, Mo: American Academy of Nursing, 29–37.

O'Hara, Patrick J. (1982). "Medical-Legal Agreement on Brain Death: An Assessment of the Uniform Determination of Death Act." *Journal of Contemporary Law* 8: 97–122.

O'Mara, Robert J. (1987). "Ethical Dilemnas with Advance Directions: Living Wills and Do Not Resuscitate Orders." *Critical Care Nursing Quarterly* 10(2): 17–28.

Omery, Anna (1989). "Values, Moral Reasoning, and Ethics." *Nursing Clinics of North America* 24(2): 499–508.

Omnibus Reconciliation Act (1990). PL No. 101-508.

O'Neill, Edward H. (1935). *A History of American Biography, 1800–1935*. Philadelphia: University of Pennsylvania Press.

Oral History (1980). New York: Columbia University Oral History Research Office.

Oral History: Evaluation Guidelines (1980). Lexington, Ky.: Oral History Association.

Parrillo, Joseph E. and Stephen M. Ayres (1984). *Major Issues in Critical Care Medicine*. Baltimore: Williams and Wilkins.

Patrick, Pamela K. (1981). *Health Care Worker Burnout: What It Is, What to Do About It*. Chicago: Blue Cross/Blue Shield Association.

Pavalko, Ronald M. (1988). *Sociology of Occupation and Professions*. 2nd ed. Itasca, Ill.: F. E. Peacock.

Pius XII (1958). "The Prolongation of Life." *The Pope Speaks* 4(4): 393–398.

Polit, Denise and Bernadette P. Hungler (1991). *Nursing Research: Principles and Methods*. 4th ed. Philadelphia: J. B. Lippincott.

Ramsey, Paul (1978). *Ethics at the Edges of Life: Medical and Legal Intersections*. New Haven, Conn.: Yale University Press.

Reigle, Juanita (1989). "Resource Allocation Decisions in Critical Care Nursing." *Nursing Clinics of North America* 24(4): 1009–1015.

Reiser, Stanley Joel (1977). "Therapeutic Choice and Moral Doubt in a Technological Age." *Daedalus* 106(1): 47–56.

Reisman, Elizabeth C. (1988). "Ethical Issues Confronting Nurses." *Nursing Clinics of North America* 23(4): 789–802.

Reverby, Susan M. (1987a). "A Caring Dilemma: Womanhood and Nursing in Historical Perspective." *Nursing Research* 36(1): 5–11.

—— (1987b). *Ordered to Care: The Dilemma of American Nursing, 1850–1945.* Cambridge: Cambridge University Press.

Roberts, Sharon L. (1986). *Behavioral Concepts and the Critically Ill Patient.* 2nd ed. Norwalk, Conn.: Appleton-Century-Crofts.

Rosenberg, Charles (1987). "Clio and Caring: An Agenda for American Historians and Nursing." *Nursing Research* 36(1): 67–68.

Rudy, Ellen B. and Donna Lee Bertram (1986). "AACN's Invitational Conference: Strategies for the Future." *Focus on Critical Care* 13(5): 44–50.

Safier, Gwendolyn (1976). "Research Q & A: Oral History." *Nursing Research* 25(5): 383–385.

Sanford, Sarah J. and Joanne M. Disch (1989). *AACN Standards for the Nursing Care of the Critically Ill.* 2nd ed. Norwalk, Conn: Appleton and Lange.

Schoffeldt, Rosella M. (1987). "Defining Nursing: An Historic Controversy." *Nursing Research* 36(1): 64–67.

Seaman, Lennie (1982). "Affective Nursing Touch." *Geriatric Nursing* 3(3): 162–164.

Seldon, Anthony and Joanna Pappworth (1983). *By Word of Mouth: "Elite" Oral History.* New York: Methuen.

Sigman, Paula (1979). "Ethical Choice in Nursing." *Advances in Nursing Science* 1(3): 37–52.

Simon, Nathan M., ed. (1980). *The Psychological Aspects of Intensive Care Nursing.* Bowie, Md.: Robert J. Brady.

Simpson, Roy L. and Lynda N. Brown (1985). "High-Touch/High-Technology Computer Applications in Nursing." *Nursing Administration Quarterly* 9(4): 62–68.

Sinclair, Vaughn (1988). "High Technology in Critical Care: Implications for Nursing's Role and Practice." *Focus on Critical Care* 15(4): 36–41.

Slemenda, Mary Beth (1983). "Brain Death Determination and Management in Children." *Critical Care Nurse* 3(3): 63–66.

Spicer, Joan G. and Mary Anne Robinson, eds. (1990). *Managing the Environment in Critical Care Nursing.* Baltimore: Williams and Wilkins.

Starr, Paul (1982). *The Social Transformation of American Medicine.* New York: Basic Books.

Stehle, Joan L. (1981). "Critical Care Nursing Stress: The Findings Revisited." *Nursing Research* 30(3): 182–186.

Stein, Janet J. (1978). *Making Medical Choices: Who is Responsible?* Boston: Houghton Mifflin.

Strauss, Anselm (1968). "The Intensive Care Unit: Its Characteristics and Social Relationships." *Nursing Clinics of North America* 3(1): 7–15.

Taylor, Lee (1968). *Occupational Sociology.* New York: Oxford University Press.

Thierer, Judith, S. Perkhus, M. L. McCracken, M. A. Reynolds, M. Aline Holmes,

B. Turton, D. S. Berkowitz, and JoAnn M. Disch, eds. (1981). *Standards for Nursing Care of the Critically Ill*. Reston, Va.: Reston Publishers.

Thomas, Lewis (1977). "On the Science and Technology of Medicine. *Daedalus* 106(1): 35–46.

—— (1983). *The Youngest Science: Notes of a Medicine Watcher*. New York: Viking Press.

Tisdale, Sallie (1986). "Swept Away by Technology." *American Journal of Nursing* 86(4): 429–430.

Tittle, Mary Beth, Linda N. Moody, and Mark P. Becker (1991). "Preliminary Development of Two Predictive Models for DNR Patients in Intensive Care." *Image* 23(3): 140–144.

Toffler, Alvin (1970). *Future Shock*. New York: Random House.

—— (1980). *The Third Wave*. New York: Morrow.

Tregarthen, Timothy (1987). "This Nursing Shortage Is Different." *Wall Street Journal*, November 11, p. 26.

Treleven, Dale E. (1981). "Oral History, Audio Technology, and the TAPE System." *International Journal of Oral History* 2(1): 26–45.

Triplett, June L. and Sara W. Arneson (1979). "The Use of Verbal and Tactile Comfort to Alleviate Distress in Young Hospitalized Children." *Research in Nursing and Health* 2(1): 17–23.

Tucker v. Lower (1972). No. 2831 (Richmond, Va. L. & Eq. Ct., May 23).

Ufford, Martin R. (1986). "Brain Death Termination of Heroic Efforts to Save Life — Who Decides?" *Washburn Law Journal* 19: 225–259.

Urban, Nancie (1988). "Responses to the Environment," In Marguerite R. Kinney, Donna R. Packa, and Sandra Dunbar, eds., *AACN's Clinical Reference for Critical Care Nursing*. New York: McGraw-Hill.

Van de Vrede, J. (1921). "The Value of the Nurse in Public Health Work in the South." *Southern Medical Journal* 14(6): 463–469.

Vanson, Rita J., Barry M. Katz, and Kathleen Krekeler (1980). "Stress Effects on Patients in Critical Care Units from Procedures Performed on Others." *Heart and Lung* 9(3): 494–497.

Veatch, Robert M. (1977). *Case Studies in Medical Ethics*. Cambridge, Mass.: Harvard University Press.

Voorman, Dorothy M. (1979). "Dedicated to a Decade of Accountability." *Heart and Lung* 8(5): 871–872.

Vreeland, Ruth and Geraldine L. Ellis (1969). "Stresses on the Nurse in an Intensive Care Unit." *Journal of the American Medical Association* 208(2): 33 2–334.

Weil, Max Harry and Robert J. Henning (1978). *Handbook of Critical Care Medicine*. Chicago: Year Book Medical Publishing.

Whitehead, Alfred N. (1931). "Introduction: On Foresight." In W. B. Donham, ed., *Business Adrift*. New York: McGraw-Hill, xi–xxix.

"Who Shall Live, Who Shall Die." *Nova*. Public Broadcasting Corporation.

Williams, William Carlos (1932/1984). *The Doctor Stories*. New York: New Directions.

Wilson, Victoria S. (1987). "Identification of Stressors Related to Patients' Psychologic Responses to the Surgical Intensive Care Unit." *Heart and Lung* 16(3): 267–273.

Winkel, Gary H. and Charles J. Holahan (1986). "The Environmental Psychology of the Hospital: Is the Cure Worse Than the Illness?" *Prevention in Human Services* 4(1–2): 11–33.

Wojcik, Jan (1978). *Muted Consent: A Casebook in Modern Medical Ethics*. West Lafayette, Ind.: Purdue University.

Wright, Susan M. (1987). "The Use of Therapeutic Touch in the Management of Pain. *Nursing Clinics of North America* 22(3): 705–714.

Wurzbach, Mary Ellen (1993). "The Dilemma of Withholding or Withdrawing Nutrition." *Image* 22(4): 226–230.

Index

University of Pennsylvania Press
Studies in Health, Illness, and Caregiving
Joan E. Lynaugh, General Editor

Barbara Bates. *Bargaining for Life: A Social History of Tuberculosis, 1876–1938.* 1992.
Michael D. Calabria and Janet Macrae, editors. Suggestions for Thought *by Florence Nightingale: Selections and Commentaries.* 1994.
Janet Golden and Charles Rosenberg. *Pictures of Health: A Photographic History of Health Care in Philadelphia.* 1991.
Anne Hudson Jones. *Images of Nurses: Perspectives from History, Art, and Literature.* 1987.
June S. Lowenberg. *Caring and Responsibility: The Crossroads Between Holistic Practice and Traditional Medicine.* 1989.
Peggy McGarrahan. *Transformation and Transcendence: Caring for HIV Patients in New York City.* 1993.
Elizabeth Norman. *Women at War: The Story of Fifty Military Nurses Who Served in Vietnam.* 1990.
Anne Opie. *There's Nobody There: Community Care of Confused Older People.* 1992.
Elizabeth Brown Pryor. *Clara Barton, Professional Angel.* 1987.
Margarete Sandelowski. *With Child in Mind: Studies of the Personal Encounter with Infertility.* 1993.
Zane Robinson Wolf. *Nurses' Work: The Sacred and The Profane.* 1988.
Jacqueline Zalumas. *Caring in Crisis: An Oral History of Critical Care Nursing.* 1994.

This book has been set in Linotron Galliard and Eras typefaces. Galliard was designed for Mergenthaler in 1978 by Matthew Carter. Galliard retains many of the features of a sixteenth-century typeface cut by Robert Granjon but has some modifications that give it a more contemporary look. Eras was designed in 1969 by Studio Hollenstein in Paris for the Wagner Typefoundry. A contemporary script-like version of a sans-serif typeface, the letters of Eras have a monotone stroke and are slightly inclined.

Printed on acid-free paper.